contents

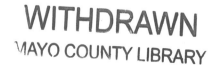

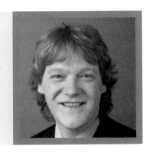

Preface

WILLIAM FAULKNER, THE AMERICAN NOVELIST, and 1950 Nobel Prize winner said in his acceptance speech, 'I believe man will not merely endure, he will prevail... he has a soul, a spirit capable of compassion and sacrifice and endurance'.

All too often in discussions about disability the focus is on the disability itself and not the person. The label 'disabled' is seen as being all encompassing, a sum total of the person, which is not true for it misses the very point that, in all walks of life, each of us are nurtured and changed by our environment, whether by family, education, career or disability. In failing to see the essence of the person, we not only do a disservice to their individuality, but we also fail to capture the totality of their being,

Within this collection, Fiona Murdoch has brought together a snapshot of many remarkable people. They are remarkable for their achievements, not just their disability. What we have on these pages is the strength and inspiration of the individual, the ability of the person to achieve their own ideals as well as leadership to others. They are remarkable for their ability to overcome the prejudices and misconceptions that society would place on their abilities.

I hope that this book will lead many others to reach for their potential to allow us to judge people on their ability, and to create a more equal society; not just speak about it. Nelson Mandela once said, 'You judge a man not because he falls but on how he gets up after he falls'. Today, at the start of the twenty-first century we should seize this opportunity to look at people firstly as individual human beings with individual rights, abilities and talents, which must be given the full opportunity to blossom.

Brian Crowley MEP

Acknowledgements

I WOULD LIKE TO ACKNOWLEDGE, first and foremost, all those who courageously agreed to be interviewed by me and without whom this book would never have come into being. The essence of *Able Lives* is the contributors and all that they have told me has had a profound impact on my being; I thank them for sharing their experiences. I am also indebted to their families, carers, teachers and others who provided additional information.

I am grateful to the good people at Veritas for making this book happen – to Director Maura Hyland, for having the faith to ask me to write this book in the first place, to my editors, Toner Quinn and Helen Carr, and also to Eimear Lynch, Eamonn Connolly and Amanda Conlon-McKenna.

Thank you to everyone else who helped me pull this book together and keep it as timely as possible. They include Cathy McGrath of the Disability Federation of Ireland, Karl Wren of the Centre for Independent Living, Rebecca Rowley of Rett Syndrome Association UK, Michael Devereux and Eamonn Duffy of the National Council for the Blind of Ireland, and Tim Kearney, national co-ordinator of L'Arche Ireland. I am also indebted to Julian Davis, Darren Kinsella, Cecilie Reid and Angela Bradley. My special thanks to Brian Crowley MEP for the Preface.

Thanks, too, to my unofficial editorial board of family and friends who generally offered their constructive and supportive comments. They are Erica Calder, Priscilla Robinson, Sylvia Lester, and my parents, Brian and Winnie Murdoch.

Thanks, also, to a number of photographers who kindly waived their copyright fee on learning that the *Able Lives* proceeds would go to three worthy causes. They are Nigel Gillis, Michael Martin, Pacemaker Press International, Belfast and Fred Hoare of *Sunday Life*.

There are many people to acknowledge, too, in regard to the CD. I am hugely grateful, of course, to the musicians and composers, all of whom generously agreed to waive their rights to royalties. I am also grateful for the help and support of Gillian Smith, Anne-Marie O'Farrell, Maeve Smith, Ann McNulty, Danusia Oslizlok, Darby Carroll, Brian McDevitt and Philippa Hogan (Four Seasons Music), Jonathan Grimes (Contemporary Music Centre of Ireland) and Mandy Byrnes (Trend Studios). Thanks, too, to Harry Bradshaw, Majella Breen, Joan Murphy and Brian O'Rourke of RTÉ. Also, to Greg McAteer and Elaine Sharkey of MCPS.

Thanks to everyone else who goes unheralded, but who has made it possible for me to achieve what I never imagined possible – compiling a book and a CD in six short months.

Introduction

THOUSANDS OF EVENTS took place throughout Europe in 2003 to celebrate the abilities and achievements of more than 37 million people with disabilities, to promote their rights and to raise awareness of the barriers they face daily in society. The European Year of People with Disabilities (EYPD) 2003 presented the opportunity both to celebrate diversity and to challenge the physical and hidden barriers that prevent people with disabilities participating fully in all aspects of society. EYPD promotes a general vision in which people with disabilities are seen as independent citizens and its focus has been to create a climate of change in which people — whether their disabilities are physical, sensory or intellectual — become more integrated into their communities.

In Ireland there are more than 350,000 people with disabilities. A press release issued by the Forum of People with Disabilities on 1 January 2003 stated that 'People with disabilities are entitled to claim 2003 as our year — a year in which our rights can no longer be ignored. It is also a year in which our identity as a distinct cultural group in Ireland should be strengthened and in which we reinforce the freedom to act to fulfil choices that we ourselves make.'

Four weeks later, speaking at the Irish launch of EYPD 2003 in the Mansion House, Dublin, Taoiseach Bertie Ahern said, 'This year provides an important opportunity for Ireland to unite with other European countries in making everyone in our community more aware of disability issues and more conscious of the rich and often underused talents that so many people with a disability possess.'

The Taoiseach's comments really hit the nail on the head because a disability in one aspect of a person's life does not mean that he/she lacks multiple abilities and talents in other areas. Too often we think of disability as inability, but that is not the case. Far from it! The stories in this book clearly demonstrate this.

The fact that 2003 was designated the European Year of People with Disabilities and that Ireland was hosting the Special Olympics prompted Veritas Publications to bring out a book to mark the occasion. It was mid-February when I received a telephone call from the Director, Maura Hyland, asking me to consider writing such a book – 'one which would contain stories of people with a disability and would talk about the ways in which they learned to live/cope with their situations'. I felt honoured to be asked and, even though I was in the middle of writing another book at the time, I knew I couldn't possibly turn down the opportunity. I love meeting different people and hearing their stories. And that's exactly what *Able Lives* is – a collection of people's stories.

It has been a great pleasure to meet each and every one of the people who appear in this book and to learn something of their lives. It has also been an enormous privilege to write up their stories to share with a wider audience. And, without exception, their stories do deserve to be heard – and to be heard widely. For they give an idea of what it is like for people with disabilities – physical and intellectual, congenital and acquired – living in Ireland today. And it is interesting to contrast the differences of their experiences.

I found it a challenge, as my editor will confirm, to keep each chapter to less than three thousand words (I could have written an entire book about each person). Most of the interviews took place in people's homes, a few occurred in people's places of work and, due to time pressures and logistical problems, two were conducted by means of long-distance telephone calls. The average length of interview was two to three hours and I used a tape-recorder on each occasion. In some cases it was appropriate to talk to others — parents, siblings, teachers and carers — in order to build up a fuller picture.

Everyone was more than willing to speak honestly and frankly about their lives — the good times and the bad, the struggles and the joys. Some wept as they recounted their struggles during difficult periods, although there was plenty of laughter, too. I don't remember encountering any bitterness; in fact, the word 'lucky' was used by a number of people in recognition of the positive aspects of their lives. I think the reason people were happy to talk so frankly, often about quite personal issues, was because they hoped that perhaps, in some way, their experiences might help others.

My only regret since finishing the book is that I didn't try to secure a ticket for the remarkable opening ceremony of the Special Olympics — surely one of the most emotionally charged events this country has ever witnessed. I did, however, enjoy a good view of the fireworks from my home in the Dublin foothills from where I was also able to see the 'Flame of Hope' burning brightly for the duration of the Games.

I have no doubt that those who read *Able Lives* will be encouraged and inspired by hearing these people's stories. I know I certainly have been. Little did I know, when I received Maura Hyland's phone call one cold February morning, how much I would be challenged, excited and changed in the course of the next six months as I met an extraordinary range of people, each with a remarkable tale to tell. Having met wheelchair users who water-ski and scuba dive and blind people who have jumped out of aeroplanes and trekked across India on an elephant, I trust that I am now less likely to equate disability with inability.

It is my firm belief that everyone who reads *Able Lives* will come away with a gratitude for their abilities, a determination to live life to the full and the inspiration to follow their dreams. But, more than that, I hope readers will be encouraged to see beyond the labels that we so often attach to people. For we need to give up on the antiquated notion that disability means inability.

One of the stated aims of EYPD 2003 was to drive progress towards achieving equal rights for people with disabilities; and at the start of the twenty-first century it is well nigh time that this happened. There is no doubt about it: it is not easy for a person with a disability living in Ireland today and it is difficult to predict the future beyond speculation and careful optimism. It is imperative that we all work towards equal rights for people with disabilities so as to make this a better place to live for everyone.

Let's hope that in years to come, we will look back on 2003 as the start of a new era – the year when Irish society began to look at people with disabilities in a new way.

Fiona Murdoch
September 2003

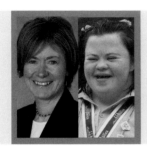

Special Olympics

... Mary Davis and Team Ireland athlete,
Lisa McNabb, share the feeling

THE ISLAND OF IRELAND HAD NEVER SEEN anything quite like it. On 13 June 2003 the Special Olympics' 'Flame of Hope', which had been lit nine days earlier in Athens, Greece, arrived at Bangor, Co. Down. From there it travelled the length and breadth of the island, with as many as one and a half million people turning out to watch it pass through their particular town or neighbourhood. On 16 June, 7,000 athletes, together with 2,000 coaches, 1,000 delegates and 11,000 family members, started pouring into Ireland's airports from 166 countries around the globe to stay with host families throughout the country. It was the start of an event the likes of which the Irish people had never witnessed before.

Who can possibly forget the extraordinary occasion of the opening ceremony of the Special Olympics World Summer Games on 21 June 2003? Croke Park became a sea of colour with the 85,000-strong crowd waving coloured flags, made by the prison community at nearby Mountjoy, while some of the most famous and widely admired people across the globe – rock musicians, politicians, and movie stars – took to the stage. Ireland's own President Mary McAleese and Taoiseach Bertie Ahern rubbed shoulders with such figures as Nelson Mandela, Mohammad Ali, Arnold Schwarzenegger and the founder of Special Olympics, Eunice Kennedy-Shriver. The pitch itself was filled with excited athletes jumping around and dancing for sheer joy – a sight to behold in itself. Can there have been a dry eye anywhere in the country as athletes, celebrities and spectators joined together in singing the wonderfully moving Special Olympics athletes' song, 'May We Never Have to Say Goodbye'?

The ten days that followed were no less extraordinary for the athletes, coaches, families, friends and spectators – not to mention the 30,000 volunteers who helped ensure the smooth running of the event. Looking back on it all now, it hardly seems a reality to Mary Davis, chief executive officer of the 2003 Games, who, together with her 280 staff members, worked 'ridiculous hours' in the months coming up to the event. 'For so long there was this frantic build-up to June 2003,' says Mary. 'We planned for all sorts of contingencies because there were so many things that could have gone wrong, but everything went to plan and all the things that might have gone wrong didn't. It was amazing! And that's why, when I look back, it seems like a dream.

'All of us who worked on the organising committee feel a huge sense of achievement at completing the project. Nothing had ever been done like it before in Ireland, so there were no templates – nothing to go by. Yet, from the time we won the bid in 1999, we were able to develop the idea, raise the necessary funding, mobilise all the people we needed and get the country behind us in the most amazing way. And, now that it's all over, I sometimes ask myself, "Did it really happen?"'

Mary first became involved in Special Olympics in 1979, when she was teaching physical education at St Michael's House, Dublin, a day-care organisation for people with intellectual disabilities. Since then she has attended every single Special Olympics World Summer Games because, finding it 'a very valuable programme', she became more and more involved – first, as a volunteer, and then in 1989 she was appointed director of Special Olympics Ireland. She held this post until 1999, when she was appointed CEO of the 2003 Special Olympics World Summer Games, a company set up for the sole purpose of organising the 2003 Games. 'We quickly adopted the slogan "One team, one goal, one chance" because, no matter what each person was doing in the organisation, we were one team working towards one goal,' she says. 'And we only had one chance to do it, so we wanted to get it right.'

Nobody could dispute that they did, indeed, 'get it right'. During the Games Mary managed to get to all but two of the sporting venues. Her personal highlights included watching athletes from Kazakhstan taking part in the long jump at Santry, seeing some of the Chinese athletes doing gymnastics 'with such amazing skill', and presenting awards after an equestrian event at Kill, Co. Kildare. 'And then, of course, the lighting of the flame at the opening ceremony was just amazing,' she says. 'I remember feeling, "We've done it! After all our toil and effort, the flame's been lit and the Games have begun." I knew the running order for the evening and I knew what was going to happen. However, it's one thing to visualise it and quite another to sit in the stadium while it's all happening around you - this vision you have has become a reality. The atmosphere was incredible. I just thought, "Wow, this is amazing!" And it was amazing!'

Lisa McNabb from Lacken, Co. Wicklow, was one of the thousands of excited athletes jumping around for sheer joy during the opening ceremony. An enthusiastic member of Team Ireland, she thoroughly enjoyed the event. 'It really was brilliant,' says twenty-three-year-old Lisa. 'There was a great atmosphere and all the people from around the world really enjoyed it. We were all up dancing and I was thrilled and happy and delighted to be there.'

Lisa and her parents, Peter and Róisín, had also attended the 1999 Special Olympics World Summer Games, which were held in North Carolina and in which Lisa competed in the softball throw and the 100 metre walk. They say, however, that the 2003 opening ceremony 'far surpassed' the 1999 event. 'We were blown away by it,' says Róisín. 'We felt really proud to be Irish.'

Lisa won a gold medal in 1999 for the softball throw and she can still remember how 'wonderful' it was when crowds of supporters lined the streets of Blessington to cheer her on her return home. Since then she has progressed from softball to shot put and from the 100-metre walk to the 400-metre walk, which she competed in at the 2003 Games. She broke her own record in the 400-metre walk and she threw her personal best in the shot put. 'Unfortunately I didn't win any medals this year, but I enjoyed doing it anyway,' she says. 'It was good fun.'

Like any dedicated sportsperson, Lisa takes her training very seriously. Under the guidance of her father, whom she describes as her 'personal trainer', she does at least half an hour of power walking each day – on the road when the weather permits, otherwise indoors on the family's treadmill. She also goes to the gym three times a week where she lifts weights and swims. 'I enjoy the training, but it's very hard work,' she says.

If Dad is away on business, her brother, David, or her sister, Leonie, ensures that she does not miss out on her training. Their father was an Olympian hopeful in his youth – he ran for his club and county – and therefore had special reason to be thrilled when Lisa qualified for Special Olympics. 'It was a great achievement altogether for her to get to the Games,' he says.

Lisa also plays basketball on Saturdays with the Blackrock Fliers at Sion Hill, Dublin – a Special Olympics club that Colm and Sheila Leech set up ten years ago, with the support of the McNabbs – and which now has approximately eighty members. Peter and Róisín reckon Lisa has 'benefited greatly' not only from participating in sport, but also from the friends she has made through the club. She often stays overnight in her friends' homes and they sometimes stay with her. Eleven members of the club took part in the 2003 Games and, when Lisa had completed her events, she enjoyed visiting other venues to watch her friends compete.

Her parents have always encouraged her to participate in a wide variety of activities and to mix with other young people. Her mum, Róisín, was a founder member of Integrated Education and enrolled Lisa in local schools – first, Lacken National School, and then Blessington Community School. 'She was offered a place in a special-needs school in Dublin when she was four, but I didn't want her going out of the area for her education,' says Róisín. 'It was a bit of a battle trying to open up the doors of mainstream schools, but we were determined. In fact, most of her friends at Blackrock Fliers also went to their local national schools.'

When she completed her secondary education Lisa attended KARE Foundation for Training and Development in Naas where she learned office skills, literacy, computer skills, advocacy and life skills. The course also included activities like horse riding, bowling, aerobics and swimming. She then completed a FÁS training course in office skills, which included one morning of work experience each week. In September 2003 she started work experience, under the supervision of KARE, in an office in Blessington; she hopes to secure employment in an office in the future.

Every Wednesday night Lisa attends a KARE-run disco in the Curragh where she meets up with her friends and her boyfriend, Conor. Lisa loves music and she cannot wait until the Blackrock Fliers' tenth anniversary dance at the end of 2003; when she's at home she loves nothing better than switching on the microphone in her bedroom and singing her heart out. When she is not busy training, socialising or singing, she catches up with her favourite television soaps – *Eastenders, Coronation Street, Neighbours* and *Home and Away*. Once or twice a year she stays for a weekend or a full week at KARE's respite house in Newbridge, which she enjoys because she gets to go on trips to the shops and the cinema. 'I love going to respite,' she says.

Lisa is keen to keep up her training and she is optimistic that she will be competing at the 2007 Special Olympics World Summer Games in Shanghai, China. 'I'm going to be there, doing the same again – the 400-

metre walk and the shot put,' she says. 'I prefer the 400-metre walk, but I'll do the shot put, too.'

Lisa knows that she must first take part in the area, regional and national games and that she must earn medals in these in order to qualify for the 2007 Games. Considering her commitment and determination, there is little doubt, however, that she will indeed be picking up plenty more medals to add to her collection (she keeps her medals in a box, which is overflowing and she says there are now too many to count). In October 2003 she started an Athletes Leadership Programme, with a view to becoming a Special Olympics basketball coach. The programme, which includes public speaking and volunteering as well as coaching skills, started with four days of training in Limerick. She was accompanied by her sister, Leonie, who acted as her mentor. Lisa looks forward to the day when she can coach basketball at the Blackrock Fliers. 'I sometimes like telling other people what to do,' she admits, 'But I do want to be friendly, too!'

That the 2003 Special Olympics World Summer Games were an outstanding success is undisputed, but Mary Davis also had a wider goal for the event. 'We wanted the Games to be very successful in terms of what they would leave behind; we believed that would be the true measure of their success,' she says. 'We hoped they would create more awareness of people with disabilities — not just here in Ireland, but around the world as well. We can be sure they have raised awareness because practically everyone on the island of Ireland is now aware of people with learning disabilities. They now know what the Special Olympics is all about and, more importantly, they know that these people are capable and able. This has happened through the various marketing and communications programmes, the schools' enrichment programme and the way we involved so many people. So you can see some of the legacies very clearly already, although it will take a while to see others.

'There will definitely be an improvement in the provision of facilities for people with learning disabilities in Ireland. As a result of the Games, we have already seen changes for the better – the government has now agreed to a rights-based legislation, which they wouldn't agree to before. I'm not saying Special Olympics was the only catalyst for this, but it was certainly one of them. And then there's the 50 million euro the government gave recently to services for people with disabilities. I think that's come as a result of the Games as well because they highlighted the whole issue of disability in a way it has never been highlighted before. As a result of that, recognition has come and some funding, which is very positive. So the Games have left behind a huge number of legacies that will transfer into more awareness of people with disabilities and a more positive life for them.

'The thing now is to keep the momentum going. Special Olympics has created awareness, but now organisations for people with disabilities have to make sure that the momentum continues. Special Olympics Ireland is a very strong programme – it's one of the strongest outside the US and that's one of the reasons we won the bid in the first place – but it can still go from strength to strength. There's still an awful lot of development left to take place.'

Mary thoroughly enjoys the company of people with learning difficulties and that's why she has spent so many years involved with Special Olympics. 'One of the great things about being around the athletes is that they are so demonstrative in the way they express their sheer excitement and joy,' she says. 'They infuse in you this sense of excitement and appreciation because they have no inhibitions. I am very appreciative of that. Like we saw in the opening ceremony, people with learning difficulties will actually get up and show their joy, whereas a lot of us are too reserved to do that. That's one of the great things I've found about being with them and that's kept me around them for the number of years that I've been involved. The volunteers experienced how infectious the athletes' enthusiasm is and they found the Games a great, great experience. They got an awful lot more out of the Games than they expected; it wasn't just about giving up a few days' work. Being around people with learning difficulties, you can't help but get a sense of joy. They teach you a lot about treating people equally and they have definitely had influences on my own life.'

Mary would love to see people with intellectual disabilities more involved in society as a whole. 'I think society would become much more enriched and enlivened and much more interesting if they actively participated in the community,' she says. 'If nothing else, that's what the Games showed. They're freer and much more open, as people, than we are and I think that's a good thing. If more people were like that, I think we'd probably get on better as a society. They're more accepting and they treat people as equals. I think that's brilliant. If we were all like that, our society would be very different.

'Going around the venues during the Games, it was astonishing to see what was going on — the way the athletes' openness was rubbing off on the volunteers and the way everybody was teaming together brilliantly. We got hundreds of letters, emails and phone calls from volunteers thanking us for giving them the opportunity to help at the Games. So you can imagine if people with learning disabilities were more involved in their communities, then their communities would be much more enriched. I think that's already happening, but it could definitely happen on a larger scale.'

The Irish people have been privileged to 'Share the Feeling', in the words of the theme for the 2003 Special Olympics World Summer Games. And that is thanks to the phenomenal amount of work Mary Davis and her team put into making the event a tremendous success. 'It's now up to every group and organisation to ensure that people with learning difficulties continue to be more involved in society,' says Mary. 'The challenge is for everybody else to take the baton and put in the effort to make sure the feeling is sustained. After all, it's there — just waiting to be tapped into.'

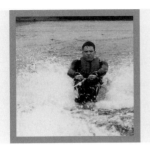

Eamonn Prunty

... a water-ski enthusiast who has set his sights on becoming world champion

ALTHOUGH HE DID NOT KNOW IT AT THE TIME, an RTÉ radio programme called *Southern View*, which went out on air one Friday afternoon in the spring of 1994, was to completely alter the life of a nine-year-old boy living in Castleknock, Co. Dublin.

For Eamonn Prunty's parents had been searching, for some time, for an activity in which their four children – Sinead, who was then twelve, and ten-year-old twins, Gavin and Oliver, as well as Eamonn – could all participate during family summer holidays. This was no easy task, since Eamonn was a wheelchair user. He was born with a spinal abnormality and, during his childhood, underwent half a dozen tendon release operations to straighten his legs.

So when one day Eamonn's mum, Carmel, heard a woman called Lil Fitzpatrick, who runs a water ski club in Carraig, Co. Cork, talking on the radio about a course she was planning to run for people with disabilities, she pricked up her ears. 'Lil was saying that she had seen some disabled water skiers, while she had been attending a water ski course abroad,' says Carmel. 'And, on returning to Ireland, she had decided to organise an open weekend for disabled water skiers.'

Lil was somewhat taken aback when Eamonn arrived for the course because she hadn't reckoned on any children turning up. However, she wasn't going to turn him away, after he had travelled all the way from Dublin, and she let him have a go. As the proverbial duck takes to water, so did the young boy from Castleknock. 'He really took to it and there was no stopping him after that,' says Carmel.

Eamonn's parents promptly made a booking to rent a cottage in Clonakilty, Co. Cork for a month, later in the summer, with the intention that all the family would try out water skiing. They did, and they all loved it. As it happened, during their holiday the European Disabled Water Ski Championships were being held nearby on the River Lee. And, even though Eamonn was fairly new to the sport, he was keen to enter. Incredibly, he came away with a bronze medal for his category in the tricks' contest.

Every year since, the Prunty family has spent their summer holidays near water – sometimes in Ireland, but also in England, Denmark, Florida and Australia. In recent years, Gavin and Oliver have become interested in wake-boarding (a water version of snow boarding), but Eamonn has stuck to the water skiing. And with good reason! His track record is remarkable, particularly considering that Eamonn, who only recently turned eighteen, has been competing against fully grown men in their twenties, thirties and forties, many of whom train full-time all year round. Apart from anything else, it is a sport that takes a huge amount of strength and stamina, as anybody who has ever tried their hand at it can testify.

There are three sections in championships – tricks, slalom and jump. During the early years of his career Eamonn concentrated on tricks, which involves performing 180 and 360 degree manoeuvres over the waves created by the speed boat that is pulling the water skier. In 1997, when he was twelve years old, Eamonn again won bronze for tricks in his category of the European championships, which were held at Lynge, Denmark. The same year he went on to win gold in tricks at the European African Middle East Disabled Championships in Aqaba, Jordan. Two years later he took gold for tricks in the under-sixteen category of the Irish National Water Ski Championships, in which he was competing against able-bodied youngsters.

In 2001 he narrowly missed getting gold for tricks at the World Disabled Water Ski Championships at Melton, Australia. After achieving joint first in the final round, he was just beaten in the run off, which meant he had to settle for silver. The following year, however, he took gold in tricks in the European African Middle East Disabled Championships, held at Schoten, Belgium. He also won his first medal for jump (bronze) and his first overall medal (also bronze).

At the Irish National Water Ski Championships in July 2003, he beat his personal best in slalom when he ran the outer course at a quarter at 40kph. The following month, at the 2003 World Disabled Water Ski Championships in Florida, he was disappointed to take fourth place in tricks and not to be placed in either the slalom or jump.

Eamonn's coach, Barry Galvin, has been Irish national able-bodied water-ski champion for the past seventeen years. What better person to coach Ireland's only competitive disabled water skier? Eamonn has had some training in other countries, including Denmark, America, Spain, and England, but he is always glad to return to Barry. 'I've trained with people all around the world, but none of them would be as good as Barry because they don't have as good an understanding,' says Eamonn. 'The only other person who has a good understanding is the Australian champion, Ray Stokes, who I've trained with three or four times.'

A training session can leave Eamonn in bouyant mood – or not – depending on how it goes. 'You get a good buzz when you do good, but it's a bad feeling when you're not skiing your best,' he says. 'If I ski well, then I'm delighted going home. The slalom is measured by speed, so it's easy to know if you're doing well: I enjoy training for it because you know exactly how you're doing. But it's hard to tell with jumps – you can tell a good jump from a bad jump, but you never know how far you've jumped in training. In competitions they use computers to measure your distance and my best so far is fourteen metres. It's hard to tell with tricks as well because in competitions the judges decide if you've done the tricks properly. Even though I'm better at tricks than slalom, I think I prefer the training for slalom because I know exactly how I'm doing.'

Eamonn's dad, John, explains how Barry Galvin and Ray Stokes take a more able-bodied strategy towards Eamonn's training than other coaches. 'Eamonn is now using able-bodied equipment rather than adapted equipment,' he says. 'Even though it is more difficult to use, it's more appropriate because it's better designed to do things at speed. It's difficult to learn on, but Eamonn's improving all the time and it will be in his favour eventually. Eamonn has trail-blazed in the equipment area because he was the first person to start using able-bodied equipment in disabled competitions. It created quite a stir when he turned up at the World's in 1999 – everyone gathered around to look at his equipment – and, since then, some of the other competitors have progressed onto using it, too. A lot of them have tried it, but there's only a few of them that has succeeded.'

Eamonn's training sessions take place on the River Lee because Barry lives in Cork. Unfortunately for Eamonn, he could not train as much as he would have liked in the run up to the 2003 World championships because he was taking his Leaving Certificate exams two months before. Apart from one week during his Easter holidays, he could not do any training until after his exams were finished in mid-June. Over the summer, he went to Cork three or four days every week, driving himself in his adapted Golf, which he bought at the end of 2002.

During his time in Dublin he certainly wasn't taking life easy. He went to the gym each day where he lifted weights, did general fitness training and swam. Eamonn, who has a small amount of movement in his legs, did not learn to swim until he was eleven years old – two years after he started water skiing. He has never been afraid of water. 'I'd been swimming with arm bands since I was a small fella,' he says, 'So I wasn't scared at all.'

It may not seem like it at first sight, but water skiing is, in fact, an extremely dangerous sport, with injuries a regular occupational hazard. Cuts and bruises are par for the course and, in the past nine years, Eamonn has also broken a leg and dislocated a knee. 'Both those injuries happened when I was doing the slalom,' he says. 'The slalom is very high risk because you can do speeds up to fifty-eight kilometres per hour and you're pulling against the boat all the time. Whatever way I twisted my leg one day, I ended up dislocating my knee. Another time I fractured my leg with the impact with which I hit the water. That was the worst because I was out of action for twelve weeks. The doctor in Cork did the best he could, but when we went to the specialist, who has operated on me since I was a baby, he said it wasn't quite right. So they broke it and reset it; I had it in plaster for another six weeks.'

The timing of this particular injury was unfortunate, given that it happened the week before the European Disabled Water Ski Championships in Milan in 2000. The result? Eamonn lost his title of European Tricks Champion because he was unable to defend it (he did win it back, though, two years later). 'It's a cruel sport,' says his father, 'Because you can train for months and, by injuring yourself just before a big event, you lose your title. There's no doubt, but it is a dangerous activity because, if you land badly on the water, it's like landing on concrete.'

Despite any misgivings he may have, John does all that he can to help his youngest son pursue the sport with which he fell in love at the age of nine. Dad has become so committed, in fact, that he has obtained planning permission for a man-made lake at Summerhill, Co. Meath, which will become the base for an Irish Aquatic Sports Centre. Given that Ireland has many natural lakes, this may seem rather a bizarre plan. However, after thorough investigation, John found it impossible to find a suitable lake where Eamonn, and other water sports enthusiasts, could practise.

'We checked out all the different lakes, but a different problem arose with each one,' he says. 'Some lakes have wildlife sanctuaries, some have big rocks in them and some don't have enough springs to feed them. We know one fella who dug his own lake in Australia and it dried up, although I don't think we need have any fear of that happening in this country! There's the Golden Falls Water Sports Centre, near Blessington, but we don't go there very often because it's not really wheelchair friendly – there are steps down to the jetty. And it's tough for Eamonn to get into the River Lee, where he does his training, because there's a very steep slope down to the river, which means, coming back up in the wheelchair, he has to zigzag up the hill.'

The idea for a man-made lake came to the Pruntys after seeing similar ones in the UK, Italy and the US. 'We'd seen man-made lakes that were built especially for the sport, so we decided to purchase some land at Summerhill, near Trim, with the ambition of establishing a training centre for everybody – able bodied and disabled,' says John. 'The lake, which was designed by Ray Stokes, will have a surface area of 11.56 acres and will be 640 metres long and an average of 65 metres wide. It's only half an hour's drive from Dublin and it's convenient to Trim, Naas and Navan. As it's situated in the middle of the country, we hope to attract people from thirty-two counties because, like the GAA and rugby, the Irish Water Ski Federation is a thirty-two county sport.'

The Pruntys have high hopes for the future of water sports in Ireland – not just for their son, but for other people with disabilities, too. 'I think the centre will be great because it has been designed with wheelchair users and blind people in mind,' says Carmel. 'It will be good that they will be able to be independent and that they won't need help to use it. A lot of wheelchair users don't think of water sports as a possibility and it would be nice if they knew that they could have a go, too: I think all wheelchair users should know that it's something they can do. If someone is a sports person before their accident or illness, then there's no reason why they shouldn't be afterwards, either.'

John and Eamonn are keen to build up a national disabled water ski team, which would include people from all over Ireland. 'Strategically, the site is well suited to that,' says John. 'We hope to be up and running by Easter 2004 and it's our plan to host the European and World Disabled Water Ski Championships. We will be bidding to host the World's in four years time, by which time we hope to have run some European events. We'd hope our reputation and the set up we'd have will be general knowledge in the sport, by then, and we'd hope to be successful in our bid.'

Eamonn, who is in his first year at the Dublin Business School, hopes to be involved in coaching at the centre. He also looks forward to the difference the lake will make to his training. 'It will mean I can train every day, which is better than doing three or four days of intense training' he says. 'It would be more spread out and I wouldn't get so tired, which is a better way to do it.'

He looks forward to seeing other people with disabilities taking up the sport because he thinks it's important for wheelchair users to find an activity that they enjoy. Looking back, Eamonn is delighted that, after spending one term at the pre-school run by the Central Remedial Clinic, his parents decided to send him to local schools – Scoil Oilibhear for primary and Castleknock Community College for secondary. Both happened to be one-storey buildings and the principals were happy to enrol a wheelchair user. Eamonn has never made an issue of his being in a wheelchair and he thinks, wherever possible, wheelchair users should attend mainstream schools. 'Just because you're in a wheelchair doesn't mean you have to be around people who are the same as you,' he says. 'It's good to mix and to find something you enjoy.'

'He's always been an adventurer,' says Carmel. 'When he was in national school he went to the Gaeltacht and climbed Dun Aengus on Inis Mór and, more recently, he climbed Croagh Patrick. He also went to swimming classes and he joined the local scouts and went camping with them. So he's a very determined spirit. He just doesn't think about the fact that he's in a wheelchair. I was quite determined, when he was little, that he wouldn't be labelled as a child with a disability; he was Eamonn. We all have our disabilities – some are visible, others aren't – and I never wanted his disability to become his identity.'

Eamonn was never teased at school and he always had a number of close friends. He is a 'huge' rugby fan and supports his local club, Coolmine Rugby Club, and often goes with his friends to international matches at Lansdowne Road. He sometimes goes away for weekends with his friends and has had 'good craic' introducing them to water skiing.

When he was a young child, his parents could not possibly have imagined what Eamonn would achieve before he reached adulthood. They certainly have good reason to be proud of him. 'Ah sure, you'd have to be – he's a star man,' says John. 'It's nice, when you go abroad, to hear the national anthem being played and to see the tricolour flying and the medal being awarded. It would make any Irish person proud, even if you weren't related to him, because it's always nice to see somebody doing well for the country, no matter what the sport. And, when it's somebody very close to you, it makes it all the sweeter.'

There can be little doubt that Eamonn will be bringing plenty more sweetness into the Prunty family in the future. Having won silver for tricks in his section of the World Disabled Water Ski Championships, he now aims to win gold in tricks, slalom and jump and, subsequently, to become overall world champion. Given his track record, his steely determination and the fact that he is competing in a sport where people often continue into their thirties and forties, it is not an impossible dream.

In fact, it is likely that sweetness will come sooner rather than later. Remember the name, Eamonn Prunty. You'll be hearing it again!

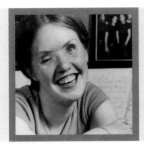

Claire Gallagher

...who played the piano in the White House seven months after she was blinded in the Omagh bombing

THE 15TH OF AUGUST 1998 began much like any other Saturday for Omagh teenager, Claire Gallagher. Her best friend, Hanora, had stayed over on the Friday night and the pair headed into town on Saturday morning to meet friends for lunch and to browse around the shops.

Their shopping was interrupted, however, when they heard there was a bomb scare. Claire and her friends were swept up with the crowds as the police started moving everyone to one end of the town. 'We kept being pushed further down,' recalls Claire. 'The police thought they were moving us further away from the bomb, whereas they were actually moving us into it.'

Once they were supposedly at a safe distance, the group of fifteen-year-old girls formed a circle and started chatting excitedly. Bomb scares in Omagh were a rare occurrence at that time and none of the girls had been caught up in one before. 'Nobody was in any real panic because nobody thought there was actually a bomb,' says Claire, 'We thought we were safe.'

The girls' excited chatter was abruptly interrupted at 3.10pm when a car bomb, planted by the Real IRA and/or Continuity IRA, suddenly exploded. Claire's life changed in an instant. One moment she was looking at her friends; the next she could see only darkness. She thought there was dust or dirt in her eyes and she called out to her friends, but nobody answered. The force of the blast had sent them flying in different directions and, when Claire stood up and began to feel her way around, she couldn't find any of them.

'I experienced an instant total blackout,' she says. 'I didn't feel anything hit me and that's why I thought it was dust or dirt in my eyes. It wasn't until a few days later that I learned a piece of metal had entered my left eye and become embedded at the top of my nose and behind my right eye. I didn't feel a thing – I had no pain – it must have been because of the shock. I never even felt the piece of metal hitting me.

'I was walking about holding my nose because I knew it was bleeding. My chin was bleeding as well – something must have hit it, too, although there was nothing embedded in it. I also realised that one of my teeth had been chipped. This fella came over and helped me sit down; he put a bandage on my eyes and then took me to hospital.'

Tyrone County Hospital was in a state of bedlam as dozens of injured people and bodies kept arriving in ambulances, cars and other vehicles. Dozens of people were wandering around in a dazed state, searching for their loved ones – not knowing if they were lying in a ward, in the morgue, in a different hospital or trapped under the rubble. 'My mum is a radiographer and she was working that day,' says Claire. 'So when one of the nurses came over to see me I said, 'Look, my mum's working in radiography. Could you let her know that I'm here?' She came over straightaway and she was so glad to see me. She was just so relieved that she knew where I was because there were so many people wandering around who didn't know where their family or friends were.'

Knowing that Claire was in town at the time of the explosion, Claire's father, Seamus, jumped in his car and headed straight for hospital. He arrived just as Claire was being taken into a side ward to have her injuries assessed. The medical staff decided she should be flown immediately by helicopter to the Royal Victoria Hospital in Belfast. 'I was lucky to have my mum and dad with me,' says Claire. 'When I arrived at the Royal I had a CAT scan and then they took me straight to theatre. I didn't know at that stage that I would never see again. I still didn't feel any pain because of the shock. In that sense, I was lucky. I don't really remember anything then until the Monday.'

While surgeons were removing the piece of embedded metal, they noticed that it had pushed Claire's right eye outwards. They realised the eye could not be saved and decided to remove it in a separate operation a week later. 'I was really upset that there was nothing they could do to save my eye,' says Claire. 'Even though I knew they had no real choice, it really upset me. When I told my friends, though, they were great about it. They said, 'Don't worry about it: we're just glad that you're still here.' My family's attitude was the same and I think that helped me to accept it.'

Claire was discharged from hospital on 30 August, but returned ten days later for yet another operation: this time, to see if the surgeons could restore any sight into her left eye. Unfortunately, their efforts were unsuccessful. 'After the surgeon came in to tell me the operation hadn't been a success, my mum said to me, "Well, what do you think?" I said, "I don't know." She said, "Well, Claire, we have two ways of looking at this. We can sit about and feel sorry for ourselves" (I said, "No"). She then said, "Right, we just have to get up and go on then." And so that's what I did.'

Claire was due to sit her GCSEs the following year and she was keen to join her classmates in Loreto Grammar School as soon as possible. Much to her annoyance, the school advised her to wait until after Halloween. 'I would have been back before that if they had have let me; I was so bored at home because all my friends were back at school.'

When she did return, Claire was already well on the way to adapting to life in darkness. 'When I came out of hospital I thought my loss of sight was going to make a huge difference with my friends. But, no, they helped me because they made me do things and they wouldn't let me sit about feeling sorry for myself. I adapted far quicker because of them. Within a couple of weeks I was going out again and doing all the normal things a fifteen-year-old does: I never let it stop me going out to discos, the cinema and into town. I did everything I would have done before I lost my sight.'

Claire began to learn braille and, after Christmas, she got a laptop computer with a speech programme, which says each letter as she types it and which can read back entire documents. She can also scan books into it. The laptop transformed her studies — both at school and, in more recent years, at university. 'Braille takes an awful long time to read and most of the material I need is on tape, so I get the tapes. If I have to read a book, I can scan it into my laptop; if I want to read a novel, I buy it on tape. The only time I use braille now is when I'm in a lift or reading signs.'

Ten months after the bomb, Claire successfully sat six GCSE exams. She then went on to study music and religious education for A-levels and in 2001 she succeeded in getting the grades she needed to study music at Queen's University Belfast. Claire loves music and there is nothing she enjoys more than playing the piano. There is no piano in the house she shares in Belfast, but she does try to make time every day to practise in the music rooms at Queen's and, at the weekends, at home in Omagh.

Claire first attended piano lessons when she was eight years old, but gave them up after a year because she was not enjoying them. Five years later she tried again with a different teacher, Bronagh Starrs, and this time she took both to the instrument and to the teacher.

Following the loss of her sight, music proved a godsend. Only a couple of days after the bomb her parents brought her keyboard into hospital. It lay untouched in a corner for a number of days until, late one evening, Claire was overtaken by a sudden urge to play. 'The keyboard had been there all week, but I hadn't bothered touching it. It was half-eleven at night when I sat up in bed playing "The Town I Loved So Well", which I'd learnt about six months before. Mum and Dad and the nurses were listening and they were all crying. At one point a nurse said, "Right, Claire, are you ready for your medicine now?" I said, "Hold on a minute. I'm on a roll!"'

Claire reckons her loss of sight has made little difference to her ability to play. 'I wouldn't have looked at the notes much before, anyway, because I'd have spent most of the time looking at the music. It took me about ten minutes to get used to playing without being able to see the notes. That was all. I love sitting down and figuring out how to play tunes for popular songs, but I also like sitting down and learning properly how to play classical pieces, although I find that a lot more demanding.'

Several months after the bomb, Claire received a phone call out of the blue from singer/song-writer Phil Coulter. He told her he was due to perform in the White House on St Patrick's Day and that he would like her to join him on stage. 'I couldn't believe it,' says Claire. 'I'd been feeling kind of numb since the accident, but I knew it would be a brilliant experience. Up until the day I wasn't too nervous, but then on the day the nerves really kicked in. It was one of the first times I'd played in public, but I did OK.'

Claire must have done more than 'OK' because, several months later, Phil Coulter again asked her to join him on stage – this time, at the Rose of Tralee festival. Since then, she has performed with him on several other occasions and in 2000 she recorded 'Carrickfergus' with him for his *Tranquillity Gold* CD. 'I played the upper part and he played the lower part. It was a wonderful experience and he was very encouraging, telling me to keep up the piano.'

Not surprisingly, Claire soon came to the attention of The Royal Irish Academy of Music in Dublin, which awarded her a scholarship to study with Maeve Smith, who was already experienced in teaching blind and visually impaired people. 'I thought it was a brilliant opportunity. I had gone back to my piano teacher in Omagh after I came out of hospital and she had managed very well, but it had been a kind of learning experience for the both of us. I hadn't done any more exam work after I lost my sight.'

Under Meave's guidance, Claire successfully sat her Grade 6 exam in 2001. She then decided to skip Grade 7. 'I wanted to get my Grade 8 out of the way before I went into the final year of my degree because I didn't want to have to work for my Grade 8 and do all my final year work at the same time. It was a bit of a jump from Grade 6 – I certainly noticed the difference in standard – but, because I did the work for two years, it wasn't too bad.'

Much to her relief, Claire passed her Grade 8 exam (with honours) in May 2003, leaving her free to concentrate on her final year studies. In her sixth year of school, Claire undertook work experience with a music therapist, which she really enjoyed and which inspired her to work towards becoming a therapist herself. 'It's the kind of thing that really interests me and it seems like a really rewarding job. I'd love to work with children because I love kids.'

Claire's own experience has taught her the power of music as therapy. 'I know when I came out of hospital that, whenever I was in a bad mood, I loved just sitting down at the piano and having a real good batter. It was amazing how good I felt afterwards!'

Five years later, the events of 15 August 1998 remain clearly imprinted on Claire's mind. 'I often have nightmares where I relive what happened or I dream about being caught up in a similar situation. In a matter of minutes my life was turned upside down. But, when I think of all the people who died in the explosion, I think I was very lucky. I also think I was lucky that I didn't see anything that day. I could hear it all – the screaming and the sirens – but it would have been worse if I had seen it as well. My friends said it was awful.'

Luck is not a word that others might use if they had experienced all that Claire has been through. After all, she was the only one of her group of friends to sustain an injury in the blast. She reckons this was because she was taller than the rest of them: now aged twenty, she stands at five foot nine and a half inches.

Nevertheless, luck is a word she often uses about herself. 'If I had lost an arm or a finger I wouldn't have been able to play the piano, so I am lucky in that way. I've also been lucky in that so many people have been there to help me. My family and my friends have been great and they've really helped me keep going: if I didn't have them, I wouldn't be where I am today.

'I'm also lucky that, because I haven't been blind since birth, I know what all my friends and my family look like. I also know, when I go shopping with my friends, if they pick out a top and say it's blue, I know what that's like. I know what everything looks like, whereas people who have been blind from birth don't. That's another thing for which I am so grateful.'

Claire has managed to maintain a great sense of humour: she jokes about the fact that she will always remember her friends as they looked when they were fifteen. 'In my mind, my friends are never going to age. And I'll always think of my brother, Christopher, and my sisters, Gemma, Elaine and Karen, as they looked in 1998. I'll always remember Karen, who's the youngest, the way she was when she was five – a little girl with piggy tails.'

When Claire returns to Omagh each Friday afternoon, she gives piano lessons to some of the neighbours' children and, being unable to tell night from day, she does not know when the pupils need the light switched on. She laughs about this. 'I start teaching at four o'clock and sometimes in the winter mum or dad have come in and said, 'Claire, would you not put the light on so the children can see?' I didn't realise they were trying to read music in the dark! Now I have to remember to ask them to tell me if they need the light on.'

As well as maintaining a great sense of humour, Claire has held onto her desire to live a full and active life. 'Losing my sight hasn't stopped me from living and people can't get over the fact that I still enjoy going to the cinema. It's not hard to follow most of the films and, if you have somebody beside you who can fill you in, there is no problem.'

Claire finds it hard to judge to what extent she has come to terms with losing her sight. 'In some ways I have come to terms with it, but in other ways I haven't. Because I've been so busy with my GCSEs, A-levels and then university and everything else, it hasn't left me with much time to think about it. I've just kind of learnt to get on with it and I suppose in that way, yes, I have dealt with it. I've learned to do things differently, but I don't know if I could say that I've really, really dealt with it. I got counselling initially, but I don't like talking to people in that kind of way and, after a while, I stopped going.'

These days Claire tries to remember what's important in her life: her family, friends and boyfriend, Ryan. 'I've got my priorities straightened out now,' she says. 'I know now that material things don't really matter. The most important thing is happiness.'

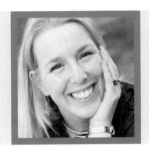

Caroline Casey

*...a visually impaired elephant-driver who
encourages others to pursue their dreams*

CAROLINE CASEY HAS LOVED ELEPHANTS for as long as she can remember. It
all started on her third birthday when her Nana and Papa gave her a squashy
orange elephant, with whom she promptly fell in love. And, thirty years later,
Ellie is still greatly treasured. For Caroline's passion for elephants continued
throughout her childhood years, spent in the south Dublin suburb of
Stillorgan, and beyond. And Ellie has since been joined by seventy other
elephants – of all shapes, sizes and colours – all of whom are equally treasured.

Following her completion of an archaeology degree at University
College Dublin in 1991, Caroline joined the ranks of young people who
take a 'gap year' to travel around the world. Twelve months of
globetrotting with her friend, Andrea Webb, did not satisfy her desire to
travel, however: it only served to whet her appetite. And, on her return to
Ireland, she remained well and truly bitten by the travel bug.

Two years later her boyfriend (now husband), Fergal Doyle, aware of
Caroline's twin passions, presented her with a copy of Mark Shand's

Travels On My Elephant. He wrote an inscription, 'For my best friend – a lover of travel and a lover of elephants'. Lapping up every word between its covers, Caroline started to imagine herself making a similar trip to the one undertaken by the author – travelling across India by elephant. She was gripped by this dream as she pored over the book – a dream which stayed with her long after she had consumed the last page.

Five years later Caroline found herself going through a rough patch at work. She was feeling negative, which wasn't like her. She is, generally, ferociously upbeat. And highly successful. With a first-class honours in her Masters from the Michael Smurfit Graduate School of Business and an Irish Management Institute award for her thesis under her belt, she had been one of only two people in her class to secure a coveted position with Andersen Consulting (now Accenture). There was a slight hitch, however. While she had ticked the visually impaired box on the application form, her future employers had never questioned her about this and she had never been particularly forthcoming about her eyesight problems. Caroline's 60/60 vision means that she is, in fact, legally blind (although she prefers to use the terms 'visually impaired' or 'partially sighted'). She can see clearly two to three feet in front of her, but only with her spectacles on; anything beyond that is 'blurry'. Caroline did not set out to deliberately mislead her employers – in truth, her incredibly upbeat outlook on life had always prevented her from admitting, even to herself, that she had a problem with her sight.

'I was in denial,' she says. 'I kidded myself that everybody else saw the same way that I did. It was only when I was told, at the age of seventeen, that I would never be able to drive that I began to realise that there was something different about me. In March 2000 my eyes really started to make me feel down – with increased responsibility at work, I felt I couldn't do my job as well as I should. I had to tell my employers that I hadn't exactly been very forthright about what I could and couldn't see. And, when I told them, they were very good. But I felt so low, having to admit that I had kind of been faking it and that I needed help. It was so difficult having to say those three words, 'I need help'. For twenty-eight years I had been trying to over-compensate because I was always so worried that people would judge me by what I couldn't do. I nearly burst with frustration because I had never learned how to ask for help in the right way.'

It was during this difficult period that Caroline told Fergal about her dream of trekking across India on an elephant. He became very quiet, later confessing that he was not very surprised – that, in some ways, he had been expecting something like that. 'He always knew I would end up doing something unconventional and he knew I had a big thing about elephants,' says Caroline. 'We'd been together six years at that stage and, in that time, he'd known me as a student, an archaeologist, a masseuse, a waitress, a landscape gardener and, finally, a management consultant. And yet he always felt I hadn't found what I was cut out for: even though I was working for one of the top companies, he knew it probably wasn't what I was best at.'

As Caroline started to plan her dream trip, she could understand Fergal's anxieties: of course it was going to be difficult for him to let his girlfriend go overseas to be with an elephant and half a dozen men in the middle of 'God-knows-where'. Naturally enough, he was concerned for her safety. Having lived with her, he was also well aware of the extent to which she 'faked' how much she could see. However, despite his understandable concerns, he was extremely supportive.

The family's response was much the same. Caroline's parents, Valerie and Gerry, sister Hillary (who has the same congenital visual impairment) and brother, Martin, were not very surprised to hear of her plans. But they, too, worried for her safety. 'They weren't entirely surprised because I've always been the most unconventional member of the family. They do worry about me – there's no doubt about it; they worry that I take too many risks (which I do), but they've never tried to stop me. They have a huge faith in my ability to face immense challenges.'

Eight months of careful planning and preparation were undertaken before Caroline finally found herself on an aeroplane bound for Delhi in

January 2001. She had arranged for an elephant, Bhadra, and a mahout (elephant driver) called Jan, to take her on a 1000km trek across southern India. The route would take her through paddy fields, jungles, game reserves, towns and cities and would include visits to a deserted palace and a Tibetan monastery.

Her introduction to Bhadra was an emotional experience. 'If there's a bit of heaven on earth, this is it,' Caroline enthused, as she stroked the elephant's trunk for the first time. The trip turned out very differently than she had imagined and, in many respects, her experience proved far tougher than Shand's. 'It was nothing like I thought it was going to be – it was so much harder – it was physically so tough and my whole romantic idea was completely smashed. Mark travelled across north-east India where they use saddles, but in southern India they ride bare back – they don't even use blankets or cushions. It was like sitting on a giant brillo pad. Mark's elephant was thirty years old, whereas mine was eighteen – a temperamental teenager – and therefore a lot more difficult to handle. Also, Mark had a good friend with him, whereas I was on my own.

'It is simply not acceptable in India for a woman to ride an elephant. People were amazed to see me and they followed me wherever I went. Physically, it was difficult on my back, my legs and my feet. It was so tough on my feet because they were constantly rubbing against the steering rope, which goes under the elephant's ears and which is used to guide the elephant: your feet literally have to push or pull at that rope.'

Caroline incurred horrific cuts to her feet as a result of the constant friction, which were made even worse when the locals decided to apply a traditional remedy of hot ash. The result? Not surprisingly, excruciatingly painful third degree burns. National Geographic, which made a documentary of the trip, refused to screen the shots of Caroline's feet because they were so horrific. Despite her agony, Caroline insisted on getting back up on Bhadra *without* bandages the day after her 'cure', which meant the steering ropes were constantly rubbing on her scars (the following day she did agree, albeit reluctantly, to wear bandages). 'No matter what happened, I was determined to prove I could do it. I was thinking, "I will do this, I will do this because I want to do this." I didn't know I had that kind of determination.'

Then, of course, there was the matter of her visual impairment. From her position on top of the elephant, she could hardly see beyond the elephant's ears. 'It was difficult because it was hard to see where I was going, so I really had to rely on Bhadra. I had this idea that, like horses and dolphins, elephants are very sensitive to people with a disability. Bhadra knew I couldn't see and she used to lead me — sometimes that was fine, but sometimes it was not so fine, especially when she started walking off the road in the direction of bananas. I have different ways of adapting — hearing, smelling and intuition — and I had to use my intuition to judge her mood.'

Halfway through the trip, Caroline suffered a devastating blow with the realisation that Jan had no intention of letting her fulfil her dream of becoming a mahout. 'It was such a disappointment when I realised he was never going to let me ride solo. To him, I was just a Western female and that was it. I got frustrated because I had worked so hard.'

Three weeks before the end of the trip, Jan decided to return to his family, leaving a second mahout, Vikram, to take his place. This was a source of great relief to Caroline — for under the tutelage of Vikram, her dream soon became a reality. In no time at all, she was up on Bhadra by herself. All the pain and hard work had paid off, after all. 'I wanted it so much because I had dreamed of it for so long. I didn't want to be seen as a failure. I am frightened of failure and, like many people, I do worry about failing. I had worked so hard to get to the point of going to India and I thought, "Well, I'm here — I'm going to give it everything I've got." It was a case of mind over matter and it was a really amazing achievement.'

Caroline is the first western woman to become a fully-fledged mahout, having condensed eighteen months' training into three months. 'There are a few things in my life I can be proud of and that is the thing that I am most proud of. I said I would do it and I did it. I can't explain what it is like living with an elephant for three months: it is the most amazing thing I have ever done in my whole life. It was a wonderful adventure.

'During the trip I learnt that the human spirit is so strong – that we have such an instinct within us to survive and to achieve, even through real pain and hell. I think when you get through adversity, whether physical or emotional, you're surprised to find such potential and strength that you never knew you had. I learnt that it is possible to achieve something, if you want it enough.'

However, the trip was not simply about fulfilling a long-harboured dream. Caroline also used it as a means of raising money for charity, founding the Aisling Project ('aisling' is the Irish word for dream) eight months before she left for India. She far surpassed her target of IR£250,000, of which £100,000 went to both the National Council for the Blind and Sight Savers International, a Sussex-based charity which treats blindness in the developing world. £50,000 went to the protection of the Asian elephant.

The fact that Caroline's own vision is non-corrective did not deter her from raising funds to ensure that others, whose sight problems are curable, could have the necessary operations. Forty-five million people in India are blind and in eighty per cent of these cases the cause is a cataract. In 2001 an operation to remove a cataract cost a mere £15 and Caroline's trip raised funds to restore the sight of an incredible six thousand people. One of the highlights of her trip had been visiting a Sight Savers screening camp where she met people who never imagined they would be able to see again. 'I saw one woman having her bandages removed and it was the most wonderful moment,' says Caroline. 'She hadn't seen anything for five years and I was so happy for her.'

In the end Caroline exceeded her fundraising target by a whopping £200,000, which she decided she would distribute to a number of other charities. That is, until she spoke to her sponsors. They were keen for her to utilise the money herself to continue the work she had already begun - highlighting the *abilities* of people with disabilities. For that had been another important aspect of the Indian trek — presenting a positive view of disability and inspiring others to live their lives to their full potential. 'I thought the trek would be a good way to capture the public's imagination regarding disability: I wanted to promote a very positive image of disability as well as encouraging other people with disabilities to get out there. It was about getting people to discuss disability in a positive way.

'I think anybody with a disability or any kind of impairment needs to feel as independent as anybody else and needs to feel included in society. When you have a disability, people tend to concentrate on the disability rather than the person: our automatic reaction is to look at what somebody can't do and to feel sorry for them. But that's not how anybody wants to be treated. I can't see well, but I can still contribute. I really believe that people with disabilities should have dreams and should be allowed to fulfil them.'

For several months after her return to Ireland, Caroline gave the matter of her future serious consideration. She had fully intended to return to Andersen's, but the media attention became quite overwhelming and, as her diary rapidly filled with speaking engagements, Caroline asked for a further three-month break from Andersen's. It was becoming clear that she was in demand because she had something different to offer. She had tried, but failed to find a charity that encapsulated what she wanted to do — promote the idea that people with disabilities have *abilities*, too. So, when her extended leave was up in September 2001 she made the decision to resign from Andersen's and to formalise The Aisling Foundation.

'The foundation has a three-pronged approach — inspiration, awareness and employment. Inspiration includes things like the elephant journey, which are intended to inspire people to look at people with disability in a very different way. Awareness refers to the fact that much of what we do is about creating awareness that everybody has ability — in other words, getting the public to understand disability in a positive way rather than a negative way. This is done through conferences, public speaking and school tours. It is also about getting people with disabilities to understand that they have a right to be whatever they want to be. Our third aim, using a work experience programme, is to increase the numbers of people with disabilities in employment in the private sector. My message to people with disabilities is, 'Just because you have a disability doesn't mean that you can't contribute and that you can't live your life. You can because everyone has ability."

Nobody could ever accuse Caroline of not taking her own advice. She continues to dream up spectacular adventures and in 2002 she took part in another 'amazing' trip – this time, going 'around the world in eighty ways' with a group of British people with disabilities. The idea was sparked by the Jules Verne novel, *Around The World In Eighty Days*, with the plan being to use eighty different forms of transport. The intrepid team of four spent three months travelling the globe, using some of the world's oldest and most unusual forms of transport – chipmunk planes, puffer boats, camels, rickshaws, steam trains, buffalo carts, vintage airplanes, jet fighters, rafts, para gliders, dump trucks and tall ships. They returned to London on 3 December – the United Nations International Day for Disabled People – where they attended a triumphal luncheon and reception in the House of Lords.

Caroline is uncertain what exactly her future holds, but one thing is definite: she will continue to live her life to the full. She has plans to set up an elephant-riding for the disabled project in India; she also hopes to spend some time living with a remote tribe in Russia. 'I have so many plans and so many dreams that I have a spaghetti-head. It's not just that there are so many things I want to do, but what I really want is to see other people come into the spotlight. I am concentrating on getting people out of the woodwork to take up the mantle.

'I think everybody wants to achieve something – no matter whether it's becoming a pop star, writing a book or going across India on an elephant – we all have something we want to do, but we don't always know how. Everyone has his or her dream and, sometimes, beginning something is the hardest thing to do. My most significant achievement has been finding the courage to start the projects I dreamed about.'

For the time being, Caroline is content to concentrate on her work with the Aisling Foundation. 'There's a lot of work that needs to be done and I really want to work at it because I love what I do. The only way you can do a job like this is to be passionate about it. The Aisling Foundation is with me in my head every hour of every day: I eat, drink and sleep the job. I now know the real sense of joy that comes from knowing what you're supposed to be doing with your life.'

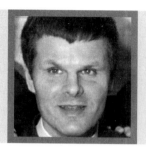

Lughaidh Ó Modhráin

... a generous musician who will never forget the time he sang for Mother Teresa

LUGHAIDH Ó MODHRÁIN IS ONE OF very few blind people currently in open employment manufacturing in Ireland. It all started in 1987 when he undertook work experience at the German-owned Wampfler factory in Baltinglass, Co. Wicklow. Impressed by the speed and accuracy displayed by Lughaidh in assembly work, his boss offered him a job as soon as his work placement was finished.

Lughaidh has never looked back. He lives in his own house in Baltinglass and, using a white cane, he makes the twenty-minute walk to work on his own each day. This was made possible thanks to Wampfler's donation a number of years ago of IR£7,500 to Wicklow County Council in order that a proper pavement could be built from the town to the factory.

When he is not at work, Lughaidh is often to be heard singing or playing his guitar. He spends weekends at his parents' home in the Curragh, Co. Kildare and often plays gigs at local venues. A committed member of the local church choir, in 1997 he was chosen to sing a solo at a Mass attended by Mother Teresa during her last visit to Dublin. Two years later he recorded an album, the proceeds of which he donated to charity.

Lughaidh also attends the local Keadeen Hotel Gym and Leisure Club. He is a keen swimmer and a member of Irish Blind Sports; he took first place in his category of the ten pin bowling competition during the organisation's annual games in 2003. He also enjoys travelling, having visited various parts of Europe and the United States.

When Lughaidh was born on 15 November 1963 it was not immediately obvious to Lughaidh Senior and Mairéad Ó Modhráin that their third son was blind because he did, in fact, respond to light. It was only seven months later, when they took him to a child specialist, who performed a series of tests, that they discovered he was visually impaired. They were told that, despite his response to light, Lughaidh was more or less blind and would have to be educated as such.

The Ó Modhráins were determined to get their hands on any literature they could about rearing a blind child. This was no easy matter. In fact, Lughaidh was two years old by the time they received much information, by which time there was another baby in the household. Síle, it turned out, was also blind. 'Nobody seemed to know anything about bringing up a blind child, but, luckily for us, the paediatrician put us in touch with a psychologist at Temple Street Children's Hospital who was to be our mentor from then on,' says Mairéad. The paediatrician gave her a small plastic chair so that she could bring Síle around the house with her all the time. 'I became an inveterate talker, explaining everything I was doing,' she says.

To this day the Ó Modhráins still do not know why two of their five children were born blind. The eldest sons, Eamonn and Cormac, see perfectly, as does the youngest sibling, Maeve. Mairéad did have German measles when she was pregnant with Lughaidh, but that does not explain why Síle should have been affected, too.

It was only a matter of time before Lughaidh Senior and Mairéad came across other parents in the area who had children with physical or intellectual disabilities, a number of whom came together to form a playgroup and special classes in Newbridge. The group became known as the Kildare Association for Rehabilitation and Education (KARE) and is still an active organisation. Lughaidh loved the playgroup, but his teacher soon found that he was mostly interested in the sounds the other children were making. 'Apparently he was very interested in sound and he was more interested in the way the teacher was saying things than in what she was saying,' says Mairéad. 'In the end the teacher told us he really needed to go to a school for the blind.'

For the next twelve months Mairéad drove Lughaidh to St Mary's School for the Blind, Merrion, one day a week and, at the age of five, he entered the school as a residential pupil. It was not a decision his parents took lightly, but they felt they really had no choice. 'Merrion was the only intake point in the country for blind children and so everyone went there,' says Mairéad. 'We went to Dublin nearly every Sunday to take him out for the afternoon and he was allowed home three times a year.'

It was customary for boys attending St Mary's to transfer to St Joseph's School for the Blind, Drumcondra, when they reached eight years of age. However, shortly before Lughaidh was due to move, Mairéad was told that he was not going to be recommended for transfer with his classmates, and instead it was suggested that he go to a school for children with intellectual disabilities.

Lughaidh's parents protested vehemently at this proposal (they knew the school in question was for severely mentally handicapped children) and decided to take him back to Temple Street for an assessment. His former psychologist was so concerned at Lughaidh's lack of progress — physically, emotionally and educationally — that she referred him to a child psychiatrist at Crumlin Children's Hospital. There the Ó Modhráins were reassured that their blind child had no educational difficulties. He reckoned Lughaidh had not been shown the differences between textures of materials, which is a basic need for a totally blind child. He told Lughaidh's parents that, without external stimulation in an unfamiliar environment, a blind child will often withdraw into himself and develop such mannerisms as rocking his body and extending his fingers. Lughaidh had developed a number of so-called 'blindisms'.

Following these consultations, Lughaidh was accepted as a pupil at St Joseph's where he made steady progress and made his First Holy Communion. He started to enjoy school. His teachers, recognising his interest in sound and music, suggested he take singing lessons at home at the weekends. A suitable teacher was found and he soon confirmed Lughaidh's singing ability, telling his parents he 'learns as good as any sighted nine-year-old'.

On hearing this, the principal of St Joseph's suggested Lughaidh should go to a school run by the Royal National Institute for the Blind (RNIB) in Northampton, England. From there Lughaidh progressed to the senior RNIB school at Condover, Shrewsbury, and then on to RNIB's Hethersett College in Surrey. He first learned to play the piano at Northampton and, during his time at Condover, he played the flute and flugel horn and joined the school brass band. It was during a work placement in a local factory near Hethersett that he discovered his interest in assembly work.

At least six other children followed the same educational route to England as Lughaidh. Some, like him, were totally blind; others were partially sighted. His younger sister, Síle, who had attended a local primary school before enrolling at St Mary's when she was eight, received her secondary education at Chorleywood College for Blind Girls, near London.

In retrospect, Lughaidh's parents feel sad that the teaching staff at St Mary's failed to discover their son's love of sound and his musical ability. However, they have been greatly relieved, ever since, to see Lughaidh thrive and their sympathies are directed towards the parents of children with disabilities for whom the educational system does not provide the means of helping them to find their children's abilities. 'Once we had recovered from the initial shock of discovering our son – and, later, a daughter – was blind, we were prepared to use every means within our power to help them cope with their handicap,' says Mairéad. 'We were not prepared, however, for the struggle we would have to get them the same educational facilities as their sighted peers.'

Lughaidh has few memories of his time at St Mary's, but he does remember how much he hated being there. 'I didn't like it and there were a few other children in the same boat as me, who didn't like it either,' he says. 'I can remember being put in a corner; I really learnt nothing there.'

Several years ago his mother, complimenting him on his success since leaving St Mary's, asked him if he recalled what might have happened that he failed to learn anything there. She was surprised by his reply. 'Every time I put my hand on the Braille machine I was slapped, so I suppose I decided to do nothing.' (Apparently that is a familiar tactic used by young children in order to avoid punishment).

On completing his education in England in 1984, Lughaidh returned to Ireland with a determination to keep up his musical interests. He joined a church folk group in Newbridge, with whom he often sang solo numbers. After four years with the group, Lughaidh joined a local family of traditional musicians – the O'Hanlons – with whom he sang and played the guitar. The group members have since gone their separate ways, but for several years now Lughaidh has been an active member of the Curragh Choir. This involves choir practice every Wednesday evening as well as singing at 11.30 Mass each Sunday morning. During the past few years he has been involved in several radio masses as well as the choir's first television Mass on RTÉ in 2003. 'The TV mass was another experience and we had to practise a lot,' he says.

In 1988, while studying singing in Dublin with Ken Shallard, Lughaidh gained fourth place in a Feis Ceoil tenor solo competition. Unfortunately, due to transport problems and his need to gain work experience, he had to give up his singing lessons. At one time he also studied the harp with Áine Ní Dhuill at the Royal Irish Academy of Music, but eventually abandoned it in favour of the guitar. For a number of years now he has performed solo gigs at various venues, which he greatly enjoys. 'I like singing, particularly to an audience,' he says. 'I like being able to give to people; that brings joy to me as well as to the audience.'

In 1995 Lughaidh produced a demo tape, a copy of which he sent to songwriter, Brendan Graham, who was very encouraging. Lughaidh later contacted the songwriter again, asking Brendan Graham if he would contribute a song for his forthcoming recording. 'If My Heart Had Wings', a song co-written with Jimmy Walsh, became the title track of a thirteen-track CD Lughaidh recorded two years later in Sulan Studios, Ballyvourney, Co. Cork. An eclectic mix of traditional and contemporary Irish songs, Lughaidh hopes this will be the first of many albums. He generously donated the profits from the first five hundred CDs to the County Kildare branch of the National Council for the Blind of Ireland. In 2003 he donated one hundred copies to the Baltinglass Committee for the Special Olympics.

Tadhg Kelleher of Sulan Studios told Lughaidh's parents that, while many people could sing, not everybody had a recording voice. Lughaidh, he said, had an excellent recording voice. Lughaidh Senior and Mairéad were delighted to hear this; they had never wanted their son's musical ability assessed any differently than if he was sighted. 'I didn't want him making an album just because he was handicapped,' says Mairéad. 'I wanted him to do it because he was capable of doing it – not because he was blind. If he wasn't deemed to be of the same standard as a sighted musician that would have put him in a different category.'

One of the songs on the album, 'Mother Teresa', was composed by Teresa O'Donnell, a songwriter from Suncroft, Co. Kildare. In 1997 Lughaidh, accompanied by Ms O'Donnell, had the great privilege of singing it in St Teresa's Church, Donore Avenue, Dublin on the occasion of Mother Teresa's last visit to Ireland. 'It was a once in a lifetime opportunity,' says Lughaidh. 'I'd say being blessed by Mother Teresa has been the highlight of my life.'

As for his work, Lughaidh is extremely grateful to his employer for giving him the opportunity to have a proper job. Wampfler has always treated him well. 'When I came back from England I did a year's work experience, thanks to Nick Carthy,' says Lughaidh. 'He gave me the chance to do work experience and, when the year was up, he gave me a job. I've been at Wampfler ever since.'

Lughaidh would like other employers to offer work placements to people with disabilities. 'I think more employers should give people the opportunity to do work experience, but I suppose other employers have different personalities to Nick,' he says. 'I probably wouldn't have got work experience if it hadn't been for him. He's dead now, unfortunately, but he was one of the best and it's not the same without him. Some people say you can't have a blind person working with dangerous machinery, but Wampfler adapted the machinery to make it safer for me. The work is quite repetitive, but there's good fun with the other staff and we listen to the radio while we work.'

Lughaidh has a computer at home, which he uses to keep in touch with his old school friends via email. He has positive memories of his teenage years and has been back to his old school at Condover a few times to meet up with teachers and friends. It was in England that Lughaidh came to grips with Braille, which he still uses, although not as much as he used to. 'I still use it for writing cards to people, but I don't use it to read books,' he says. 'My computer has a speech programme and I have a scanner, which I use to read books. I like books, but I think I prefer the computer now.'

His sister, Síle, who earned a PhD in computer music from Stanford University, is currently undertaking research into haptics technology, which involves extending the experience of computers to include not only vision and sound, but also touch. This will be of great benefit to blind people. She is the principal research scientist heading up the palpable machines group at Media Lab Europe, the Dublin-based European research partner of the Massachusetts Institute of Technology's Media Lab. Also a keen musician, Síle has sung, at various times, with the RTÉ Philharmonic Choir, the Irish Youth Choir and the BBC Symphony Chorus.

There is no doubt about it, but Lughaidh and Síle are lucky that their parents have always sought the best for them and encouraged them to pursue their various interests. Mairéad and Lughaidh Senior have always believed that blind people should be encouraged to lead independent lives. 'I've never thought the blind should be objects of charity,' says Mairéad. 'I've always felt that they had as much right to independence as anybody else and that they must learn to make it themselves. Our children's blindness was a challenge to overcome, but never at the expense of as normal an upbringing as their sighted siblings.'

Looking back, Lughaidh finds he is more accepting of his blindness now than he was as a child. 'When I was small I didn't quite accept my blindness, but it doesn't bother me as much now,' he says. 'I don't think about it as much as I used to.'

Whatever happens in the future, music is certain to feature largely in Lughaidh's life. 'I hope to continue working at Wampfler, but at least if my job ever fell through, I'd have my music,' he says. 'In the long term I'd like to make more albums, but I need to get access to a studio and find somebody to work with me. If I had somebody to help me produce another album, it would be great.

'I think the main thing is just to keep up my singing,' he adds. 'That's my main aim for the future.'

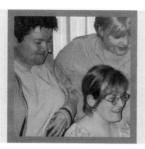

Jeanette Craig
and Hayley Osbourne

*... who overcame obstacles to enter third-level
education*

JEANETTE CRAIG AND HAYLEY OSBOURNE live in a hostel in Carrickfergus, Co. Antrim. Three days a week they attend classes at the nearby East Antrim Institute of Further and Higher Education (EAIFHE) and two days a week they are involved in work placements.

Jeanette's work placement is in the hostel kitchen, where she washes dishes and mops the floors of the kitchen and food store; Hayley's is in the kitchen of the University of Ulster at Jordanstown where she does similar work to Jeanette. Both enjoy their placements, even though they receive no payment.

They also enjoy the cookery and personal grooming classes they attend at EAIFHE, where they learn valuable skills. In personal grooming they learn how to wash and dry people's hair, which in theory means that, at some stage in the future, they should be able to secure employment in a hairdressing salon. In practice, however, this is unlikely to happen.

When they are not on work placement or attending classes at EAIFHE, both women are to be found in Hawthorne's Day Care Centre, which is situated next to the hostel. There they spend some of their time folding boxes for contract work. They do not get paid for this either.

Despite the fact that they are both well able to work, the fact is that neither Jeanette nor Hayley is likely to get a salaried job. Ever.

If they were children in some country in the developing world, this would be called exploitation. But they are adults in a supposedly developed country, so how can this be happening? The answer is quite simple: Jeanette and Hayley have intellectual disabilities and, as such, are unlikely ever to be taken on by an employer.

It is a situation that the co-ordinator for people with intellectual and physical disabilities at EAIFHE, Deirdre Kelly, finds unsatisfactory. 'I would see having a job as a right for these people,' she says. 'We've been teaching students with learning disabilities for sixteen years and, in that time, only three people have gone on to get work (they got packing jobs in factories). People like Hayley and Jeanette are doing courses and work placements that are valuable in developing their skills, but the fact of the matter is that they will probably never get full-time employment. We now have four hundred students with learning disabilities on our books who are gaining employability skills, but very, very few will actually go on to employment.'

Deirdre feels the root of the problem lies in an inflexible system. 'The big problem is the benefits trap,' she says. 'In order to work they have to give up their benefits and, if they get a factory job, they are not really any better off. Often the benefits are part of the family income and, if you have someone living at home getting disability benefit, there could be a mobility component and a care component for someone looking after that person. So helping that person to become more independent can mitigate against you because the more independent they become, the more likelihood there is of having the benefits reduced. It's a very difficult trap for some people.'

Deirdre would love to see the adoption of a more flexible approach. 'I'd like to see something done about benefits to help people live more independently,' she says. 'Maybe they could come in and out of work — maybe try a job for a few months and then, if it doesn't work out, come back into the benefits system again, without having lost their entitlements. The problem is that once you say you're fit to work, that's you fit to work for the rest of your life: now, if you try out a job and it doesn't work out, you aren't guaranteed a place back in the system. I think we need more flexibility.'

Deirdre sees no reason why people like Hayley and Jeanette should not be in paid employment. 'If there were proper supported opportunities for employment, there's no reason why people with learning disabilities couldn't be working in a proper environment. But, the way the system works at the moment, there isn't the flexibility for that. There's a funding issue here, of course. If we were doing better in society we would maybe provide someone to train them up for a few months to do a particular job and come back and visit them from time to time. It would be an investment.'

Deirdre is in no doubt that society, as a whole, would benefit from the presence of people with intellectual disabilities in the workforce. 'Like any group of people, there's a wealth of talent there — there are different sorts of talents — and people with learning difficulties have an awful lot of contributions they could be making to society. I think it's important that people with intellectual disabilities become more involved in society. It's a human rights issue.'

An important place to start, she reckons, is to listen to what these people want. 'They are as entitled as anyone else to have their voices heard and we have to be better at listening to their voices and giving them opportunities to say how they feel about things. We need to get better at finding out what kinds of services they want. And I think we have to be careful not to put words into their mouths because, with someone with a learning disability, it can be very easy to get them to say what you want them to say. It really, really can.'

Deirdre's own background lies in primary school teaching, although she started teaching adult literacy classes in EAIFHE in 1987. A couple of women with learning disabilities from a local day care centre heard about these classes and asked if they could attend. As it turned out, they had very poor literacy skills. As a result of listening to them, Deirdre discovered that these women were interested in attending other classes, too. Rather than trying to slot them into classes with sixteen- and seventeen-year-olds, the institute decided to start up classes especially for them. One of their parents came up with the name Horizons for this programme since the whole idea was to broaden the experiences of the participants.

Horizons has been up and running for fourteen years now and attracts people from a variety of day care centres in County Antrim. The programme has gradually broadened over the years to include such diverse subjects as line dancing, physical education, woodwork, brickwork, gardening, art and computers as well as basic skills in English and maths and, of course, cookery and personal grooming. 'Really, the whole range of subjects on offer at EAIFHE is available, at an appropriate level, to people with learning difficulties,' says Deirdre.

Students choose whichever subjects interest them. 'I'm looking forward to doing more personal grooming classes next year,' says Jeanette, who has attended EAIFHE for the last eight years. 'We learn to put make-up on as well as learning to wash and dry hair. We also do some writing: today we were writing about the dangers of hair dryers. I like college. The only thing I don't like is that, some days, you can't get in because there's that big a crowd of young ones hanging around.'

Along with the other students, Jeanette and Hayley always look forward to presentation night, which is held in June each year. The occasion affords them the chance to dress up and put to good use the make-up skills they have learned in their personal grooming classes. 'I like to go to college to get my certificate at prize night,' says Hayley. 'You have to wait to hear your name called out and then you have to go up and shake hands with the guest and the director and then you get your certificate.'

Hayley is one of two students with learning disabilities who are members of a newly-formed focus group, which was set up to look at policies for people with disabilities in the institute. 'The focus group allows the learners to say how the services impact them, so we can assess the impact of any policy on them,' says Deirdre. 'We also have people representing wheelchair users and people who are visually impaired. It's to try and give them a voice. Their link worker comes with them to the meetings to help them understand what's going on and to help them make their viewpoint heard.'

Deirdre, who is currently studying for a Masters in Lifelong Learning at Queen's University Belfast, believes attending college does wonders for people with intellectual disabilities. 'As well as broadening their horizons and developing their personal skills by giving them a variety of experiences, they are also gaining important social skills,' she says. 'They learn how to behave appropriately: when you're stuck in a day centre all day, you don't learn how to relate to different types of people. You see their confidence and their assertiveness increasing because they're getting the same opportunities as other people. They like the idea of being students – they like that description of themselves – and, like the other students, they really like going to the canteen.

'It's good, too, for the other students to see that these people are a part of the community – that they are out and about, that they do come to college and that they're not going to go away. The students are fine – there has never been any problems with name-calling. Occasionally we've had complaints about staring, but that's all.'

What has Deirdre learnt from her sixteen years' involvement with people with intellectual disabilities? 'I have learnt that they're a group of very different people and that you must listen to what they need rather than giving them what you think they need. It has certainly made me sure to listen more to what people say. Working with them has helped improve my communication skills — I'm better now at simplifying things and speaking to them in a language that they understand.'

Apart from the annual nightmare of drawing up timetables, the biggest challenge Deirdre faces is finding suitable tutors. 'Not everybody is suited to this kind of work: some people are frightened of people with disability because they feel uncomfortable and inadequate around them. But I think if you're good with people and, if you take the time, you can communicate with anybody. Some people are brilliant and, if I had those people multiplied by three, it would be great!'

Eithne Agnew has been teaching computer classes at EAIFHE for ten years, but it is only in the past twelve months that she has taught students with learning disabilities. Her lack of relevant training meant she was reluctant to do this at first, but in the end she agreed to 'give it a go'. It has proved a rewarding, even life-changing, experience. 'I don't know how much they've learned,' she says, modestly, 'But they're happy and I'm happy. And we're all learning.'

She reckons she learns something new each week from her students with learning disabilities. 'I've related so many stories to my own children — things I've learnt from the learners,' she says. 'I've a card stuck on the fridge at home that one of them took the time to make me. The day she gave it to me, I just felt so humble that she would do that for me, and I asked myself, "Why can't I accept what others do for me with the same humility and gratitude? Is it because I feel that it cost her something to make the card — that it took her time?"

'I still have to work out the answer to that, but I do know the joy it gives me to have that card. Perhaps it's because our expectations of each other are, so often, very high and it's taken that card to make me go back and appreciate the little things again. People with learning disabilities celebrate — even the little things — with so much enthusiasm and joy. They've really made me stop and think; they've given me a completely different view of life.'

Eithne has been hugely impressed by the way they share wholeheartedly in each other's joys and successes. The joyous way in which they sing 'Happy Birthday' to each other is just one example. 'There's a different – I suppose, special – way they celebrate with each other,' she says. 'It's always a learning experience for me and, so many times, I just feel I would love to have that freedom to be so free to celebrate with other people. I think we've lost that a bit in society.'

When Eithne discovered that one class member, Grant Wilson, was going to swim in the Special Olympics, she found his photograph on the internet to show the other students. 'I gathered them all around and brought it up on the screen to show them and, when they saw his photograph on the computer, they really celebrated with him. I thought the way they responded was so refreshing; they went up to him and shook his hand and congratulated him. They seem to be able to celebrate each other's achievements without any sense of jealousy.'

Another time, when Christopher McKinstry told Eithne he got an award for snooker, she was taken aback by his response when she said, 'That's great. You must be good at snooker.' He replied, 'Yes, I am.' Eithne says, 'If somebody said that to us we would probably play it down by saying something like, "Ach no, I'm not really". I found his honesty very refreshing: he was simply recognising that he was good at something.'

Eithne finds her students with learning disabilities are always extremely grateful. 'With the other students it's a battle of wits because only two in a whole class might be interested in learning, whereas the adults with learning difficulties are so grateful to learn any little thing. Some of them do very well and it's surprising just what they can do. The last few weeks I've been getting them to type out different poems. They enjoy doing that, but if you did the same poems with seventeen-year-olds, they'd just be so sarcastic. The attitude of the adults with learning disabilities is so different: you can see, when you do something for them, they're so appreciative. And that makes me feel good.'

Eithne has been touched by how affectionate some of her students with learning disabilities are, particularly the women. 'They are very free: they come up and kiss me and hug me and say, 'I love you, Eithne.' That's not something I've been used to, but I love it! I think it's mega! I suppose, in some ways, I feel quite humble that they feel they have the freedom to kiss me and hug me. I feel that they identify something in me that allows them to do that – they know they're not going to be rejected. It makes me wonder why I cannot have that same kind of openness all the time. What are the barriers that we put up with each other?'

Has the experience of working with people with learning difficulties changed Eithne? 'Totally. Because of the warm welcome they have given me and because of the lessons I have learned from them, like being appreciative of the little things in life and acknowledging the gifts that you have. They have also reminded me that what you get back from people depends on what you give out.'

She is in no doubt that the students do benefit from attending classes in EAIFHE. 'They see themselves as doing something that everyone else is doing. There's a level of intellect people with special needs can arrive at – it might take them longer, but they do arrive there. For them, I think it's important.'

Like Deirdre, Eithne would like to see people with intellectual disabilities more involved in mainstream society. 'We're living in a very materialistic society and I think we've lost some things, like welcoming each other and celebrating with each other. People with learning disabilities express their feelings very freely: they'll come into the classroom and say, 'I'm happy today', 'I'm sad today' or 'I really love you'. They have this total freedom. What does that say about us? We accept that type of honesty from people who society says are 'broken', yet those of us who are not 'broken' cannot be that honest with each other.

'I think the more we've got materially, the more we have to protect and the more insular we become. We do that with our feelings as well because we don't even trust each other with our true feelings. We don't allow each other to be less than perfect.'

There is no doubt in Eithne's mind that society would benefit from greater involvement of people with intellectual disabilities. 'The joy that people with learning difficulties have and the freedom they have to express their feelings is remarkable. I think we could learn a lot from them.'

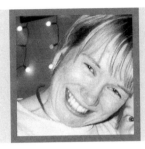

Siobhán Keane

... a passionate pianist, enthusiastic educator and spirited scuba-diver

SIOBHÁN KEANE IS A PASSIONATE PIANIST whose many interests include education and scuba diving. As well as a teaching qualification, she holds a BA in music and Irish, a Masters in Education from St Patrick's Teacher Training College, Dublin and a Masters in Music Education from Columbia University, New York. She also has a Licentiate piano teaching diploma from the Royal Irish Academy of Music. And then there's the scuba diver's licence she received in July 2003!

A primary school teacher in Dublin for almost twenty years now, Siobhán can remember the early days of her career when she had so much energy and enthusiasm that, when she came home from work, she would sit down and play the piano for four hours. Just for fun!

While she still has a great zest for life, Siobhán has never enjoyed that same level of energy since she was involved in an accident one Friday evening in April 1994. A truck driver omitted to signal his intention to turn left and Siobhán, who was cycling alongside the vehicle at the time, ended up under its wheels. She sustained a spinal injury and was left without any feeling or movement in her legs.

She remembers every detail of the accident, but wisely chooses not to dwell on it, having 'moved on' since then. She does not dwell on the fact that she can no longer cycle, even though her bicycle had been her primary means of transport (she learnt to drive, albeit reluctantly, some months after her accident). Neither does she dwell on the fact that she cannot enjoy the full capacity of the piano, since she is unable to use the foot pedals.

It was during the three weeks following the accident, while she was recovering in the Mater Hospital, that she was told she would never walk again. She was moved to the National Rehabilitation Hospital in Dún Laoghaire where, as she was grappling to come to terms with this devastating news, she received a 'really empowering' piece of advice from the late Dr Joseph Groocock, who was a music lecturer at Trinity College Dublin at that time. 'While you've got your mind, you've got everything,' he told her.

Groocock, who was a Bach scholar, suggested various harmony and counterpoint exercises that Siobhán could carry out on her keyboard while she was in hospital. She followed his advice and found that writing music was a terrific means of keeping her mind active. She also found herself playing a great deal of Bach because, since he composed for the harpsichord (which has no pedals) his compositions could be played on the keyboard. And Siobhán knew that, when she was finally discharged from hospital, she would only be able to play her piano without using the pedals.

Fortunately, Bach had been one of Siobhán's favourite composers for many years – a fact that, perhaps, went a tiny part of the way towards easing the tremendous blow of no longer being able to appreciate the full mechanics of the piano. 'Bach was a genius – he was such a prolific composer,' says Siobhán. 'There was nothing affected about him; he loved life and he lived it to the full.'

Although she would be too modest to say so, Siobhán has certainly followed in the footsteps of her hero in that regard. She, too, believes in living life to the full. While it took some time for her to adapt to using a wheelchair, it certainly never destroyed her enthusiasm for life. Within two months of leaving hospital she returned to her job teaching in a primary school in Dublin's north inner city where she was assigned a classroom on the ground floor. The children loved opening doors for her and helping her in any way they could, with the result that teacher and pupils built up a particularly good rapport. 'The children were fantastic; they were delighted to help,' remembers Siobhán. 'It made them feel so important.'

Siobhán gradually adapted to playing the piano without using the pedals and in 1997 she performed with Danusia Oslizlok in the Peppercanister Church to raise money for L'Arche, an organisation which involves volunteer assistants and people with intellectual disabilities living alongside each other in small communities. She started to enter various competitions, as she had always done, and was delighted to win the Benson Cup for playing compositions by Bach at the Dublin Feis Ceoil in 1999. She also continued to give recitals at various Dublin venues, including the Royal Irish Academy of Music and the Royal Hospital Kilmainham.

Somewhat frustrated with the limited repertoire of pieces that she could now play, Siobhán asked composer Philip Martin to write a piano piece that would not require the use of pedals. 'I was looking for something that was a bit different and Philip jumped at my request,' she says. 'I suppose he saw it as a challenge'. He obliged by writing not just one piece, but three, which he entitled *A Suite For Siobhán*. She performed these pieces, which were officially commissioned by the Contemporary Music Centre of Ireland, for the Contemporary Irish Music Cup at the Dublin Feis Ceoil in 2000.

Philip Martin wrote one of the test pieces for the semi-final round of the AXA International Piano Competition held in Dublin in May

2003. Siobhán went to listen to as many of the pianists taking part in the event at the National Concert Hall as she could. 'It was phenomenal,' she says. Siobhán herself competed in the Irish round of the second such event, then known as the GPA International Piano Competition, in 1991.

While she does not have the energy that she used to have, Siobhán finds that she wants to preserve what energy she does have for a wider variety of interests than before. Prior to her accident the piano had been very much her primary focus. She now plays the fiddle more than she used to and, in recent years, she has taken part in the Willie Clancy Summer School in Milltown Malbay, Co. Clare and Scoil Acla in Achill, Co. Mayo. These summer schools offer a wonderful outlet for all ages to share music together.

Her interests now extend far beyond the confines of music and she has become something of an adventurer. When, fifteen months after her accident, she went to visit her sister, Bláithín, in Australia she did not think twice when her brother-in-law, Ian McCrimmon-Stobbie, offered to take her for a spin on the back of his motorbike (he duck-taped her feet to the footrests to prevent her falling off). She also seized the opportunity to try her hand at water-skiing.

On her return to Ireland she decided to investigate scuba diving and found she loved the sensation of being in the water. 'There is an incredible freedom because your wheelchair isn't attached to you,' she says. 'It's very liberating. The great thing is that you don't have to use your legs — it's enough to use your upper body to swim.'

Siobhán dives with the Lir Sub Aqua Club, which is one of the many clubs of the Irish Underwater Council. During the winter months she attends their weekly training sessions in the swimming pool at the Central Remedial Clinic in Clontarf. The rest of the year the club dives off Howth, Sandycove and Dun Laoghaire as well as making weekend trips to places like Kenmare, Achill, Sligo and Donegal. Siobhán loves the social side of the club. 'You're there in a pair of wellies and a wetsuit and you look awful, but the lovely thing is it doesn't matter because you feel so invigorated,' she says. 'After a dive we always hit the pub – I'm not a drinker, but it's sociable and it's a great opportunity to chill out.'

Since she has benefited so much from her foray into scuba diving, Siobhán would urge anyone else who finds themselves injured or in a wheelchair, following an accident, to seek out some kind of hobby. 'I think it's so important to get back into life and not to retreat into yourself, which can leave you feeling isolated,' she says. 'It's important to get out into the big picture, to push out the boundaries and get involved with people. Once you are involved in activities you enjoy you will remain mentally healthy and, when you're mentally healthy, you will be physically healthy.

'The big danger, for anyone who has a physical disability or who finds themselves in a challenging situation, is that if you get depressed you will stop looking after yourself. It's essential to keep mentally well and to find physical outlets because it's important to feel good about yourself. Although I certainly don't think I have the balance right, at least I am trying to maintain a healthy existence.

'When you've had an accident your whole life direction can be really thrown off kilter and it's difficult not to stagnate. I do think it's important for people to continue to strive to better themselves – perhaps pursuing studies for work or leisure. As a teacher, I really believe that education is important.'

Siobhán has fond memories of her school days – firstly in Castlebar, Co. Mayo, where she lived until she was eleven – and then in Kilkenny, where her family moved in 1974. Her last year of primary schooling was spent at St Canice's National School, Kilkenny, which happened to be one of the few primary schools in the country to have a full orchestra. 'There were violins stacked all along the walls of the school and there was a hiring system,' remembers Siobhán. 'It was a thriving, vibrant set up.'

Siobhán was already steeped in music because she had been born into a musical family – her mother, Mary, is a piano teacher and her father, Joe, was 'a fine singer'. Many an evening saw the Keane family gathered around the piano, singing Percy French songs. Siobhán started formal piano lessons at the age of seven (her mother was too busy to teach her since Siobhán was the eldest of six children). 'I really loved the piano from day one,' recalls Siobhán. 'I took to it straightaway.'

It was during her second level years – spent at Loreto Convent, Kilkenny – that Siobhán first considered pursuing a career in music. However, although she had successfully completed her Grade Eight exam in fifth year, the careers guidance teacher cautioned her, suggesting she apply to do primary school teaching. 'At least you're guaranteed a job,' she advised. 'You can always pursue music afterwards.'

Looking back now, Siobhán is grateful for that piece of advice. She was very interested in teaching, anyhow, and applied to Carysfort College. After gaining her teaching qualification, she taught for a year and then signed up at University College Dublin to study music, taking Irish as a second subject. During these years in Dublin she also pursued her piano studies with pianist Anthony Byrne.

After graduating from UCD, she taught for another year before deciding to further her musical studies – this time, on the far side of the Atlantic. In 1988 she moved to New York where she studied for a Masters in Music Education at Teachers College, Columbia University. 'It was a wonderful course because you could design your own programme,' she says. 'I studied violin pedagogy, choral conducting and all kinds of aspects of music teaching. I also studied piano privately for a year at the Juilliard School and, during my second year, I worked with a teacher at the Manhattan School of Music. I also had the opportunity to go to two wonderful summer schools in Aspen, Colorado, and Victoria, Canada, where I took piano lessons with a number of different teachers, including Hungarian pianist and pedagogue Bela Siki and Robin Wood, director of the Victoria Conservatory of Music.'

On her return to Dublin, Siobhán spent three years working on a pilot scheme in the inner city initiated by the Department of Education. She was one of thirty home-school liaison teachers appointed and worked with five inner city schools. 'It was a wonderful philosophy designed to help parents see the value of education,' says Siobhán. 'The whole idea was to open up schools to the community and to make them a resource for the community. And so I became involved in setting up various courses, including a music class for parents and their young children.'

Around that time Siobhán also set up the Inner City Children's Choir, which performed in St Canice's Cathedral during the Kilkenny Arts Festival in 1992. She was subsequently invited onto the festival's music committee and, for the next six years, was involved in running children's workshops at the annual event. 'We had workshops in art, drama, music and dance movement. Children were exposed to all the various art forms and participated for a week, benefiting from a process focused approach.'

Siobhán was back in the classroom, teaching fifth and sixth class, when she had her horrific accident in April 1994. She had been living in a bedsit in Rathmines and, while she was in hospital, her family and friends, knowing there was no way she could return to live in such a small space, looked around for suitable accommodation. In the end, her parents found a spacious enough ground floor apartment in Sandymount, where Siobhán lives to this day. For the first four years her 'hugely supportive' younger sister, Bríd, shared the apartment with her. Siobhán enjoys the 'village mentality' of the area and the fact that, unlike many other parts of the city, most of the pavements are 'lipped'. She also likes being near the sea.

Two fundraising concerts were held in 1995 to raise money for Siobhán to purchase an adapted car. The first was organised by Paddy Sommerville, a retired teacher, the second by Canteoirí Avondale, a choir that Siobhán used to sing with. After taking driving lessons, she returned to teaching on 31 March 1995, less than a year after her accident. Although she loved the pupils of the inner-city school where she had taught for fifteen years, she knew that in many ways life would be easier for her at a wheelchair-friendly school. Four years later, when Siobhán was offered a teaching post in the primary school attached to the Central Remedial Clinic (CRC), she didn't have to think twice before accepting it. 'The school has automatic doors and I can't describe the beauty of that,' she says. 'The fact that the whole building is wheelchair accessible is so lovely because it makes life that much easier. There's plenty of space to manoeuvre and that's very important for my mental and physical wellbeing.

'Initially, I found teaching at the CRC a big challenge because some of the pupils are non-verbal, so there's a huge emphasis on communication skills for teacher and pupils. Of course, music is a hugely powerful communicating tool and that was a great link for me straightaway. It didn't take long to realise that these children were like any other – they had the same needs of wanting to have fun and wanting to make friends.'

Siobhán has been interested, for many years, in rhythm and movement and in 1996 she went to the Dalcroze Institute of the Juilliard School, New York where she spent three weeks studying the pedagogy of the Swiss music educator, Emile Jaques Dalcroze. In the early twentieth century, Dalcroze developed a series of exercises entitled 'eurythmics'. 'It is all about enabling people to feel rhythm in their bodies,' says Siobhán, 'The whole premise is that, before children are presented with musical instruments, they should receive training in their bodies.'

Since then she has passed on this knowledge to dozens of primary school teachers throughout Ireland and in July 2002 she returned to the US to further develop her skills. She is involved with Fuaim, a voluntary organisation set up in 1997 to promote music education in primary schools. 'Our goal is to bring music to every child in the country via their regular classroom teacher,' she says. 'We run a large number of courses on different aspects of music teaching.'

Incredibly, Siobhán has also found time to pursue a Masters in Education, which she was awarded by St Patrick's College of Education in 2000. It was based on a 'Write an Opera' project, which she carried out with pupils with physical and learning disabilities – the children wrote, composed and performed their own opera. 'Sometimes opera is seen as something elitist, but really an opera is simply a story with music,' says Siobhán. 'The children called the opera, *Friends Care About Each Other*, and the whole beauty of the project was that its focus was very much on the process, not the end product.'

At this point in her life – she has recently turned forty – Siobhán sees herself first and foremost as a music educator. 'I love music and its ability to communicate,' she says. 'And it's my love of music and people that's the driving force for me. There's so much that can be done within the regular primary school, without it being formal or intense.

'Everybody should have exposure to the joy of music-making, singing and playing instruments,' she adds. 'Music shouldn't be an elite skill; it should be for everybody.'

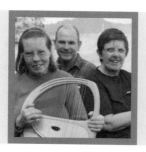

The Camphill
Community Celtic Lyre
Orchestra

... which includes sixty people with intellectual disabilities and which has performed in the National Concert Hall

HAVE YOU HEARD THE ONE ABOUT the Scotsman, the Englishman and the Irishman? Well, the Scotsman, on hearing the Englishman play the lyre, came up with the idea to build a lyre which would be suitable for people with intellectual disabilities to make and to play. The result was that the Irishman designed the instrument, the Scotsman built it and the Englishman taught one hundred people, including sixty with intellectual disabilities, how to play the instrument.

Within two years of the first instrument being designed by Irishman, Sam Irwin, and built by Scotsman, Clifford Paterson, the Camphill Community Celtic Lyre Orchestra, conducted by Englishman, John Billing, played to a packed audience at Belfast's most prestigious venue – the Waterfront Hall. They received rapturous applause and a standing ovation. Ten months later, on 19 November 2002, they performed in the National Concert Hall in Dublin where they were joined on stage by world-renowned musicians Phil Coulter and Brendan Monaghan as well as John Sheahan of the Dubliners and Lynn Hilary of Anúna. The Irish president, Mary McAleese, attended the concert and, afterwards, congratulated members of the orchestra on their remarkable achievement.

Incredible as it may sound, this is not a joke; it is an astounding fact. A fact which the brains behind it all, Clifford Paterson, can hardly believe himself. He shakes his head in amazement when he considers how quickly the project has mushroomed. It all started when he attended a concert given by John Billing, the world's only professional lyre player, at the Camphill community in Mourne Grange in 1999. Clifford had moved there from his native Scotland two years earlier. Situated in a fabulous location on the lower slopes of the Mourne mountains, near Kilkeel, Co. Down, the Mourne Grange community consists of eighty volunteers who live and work alongside sixty people with intellectual disabilities.

Following the John Billing concert, Clifford determined to find someone to help him design a Celtic lyre that could be manufactured at the Camphill workshop, which at that time was producing garden furniture. He contacted Sam Irwin, a Bangor man who makes highly-crafted musical instruments, and, together, they created the Celtic lyre which won first prize at the Royal Dublin Society National Craft Awards in 2001.

'A lot of people have heard of the lyre from ancient Greece,' says Clifford. 'It's a very angelic instrument, which connects us with the spirit world. In the 1920s the philosopher and educator Rudolf Steiner, who is one of the spiritual leaders of the Camphill communities, indicated that the lyre was a good instrument for people with special needs because of its healing, meditative sound. As a result of his inspiration, the first modern lyre was made in Germany in 1926.

'The difference between a Celtic lyre and any other lyre lies in its shape and design — it is more curved than the German lyre, which is quite functional. There had been no Celtic lyre in existence since, maybe, the tenth century. Resembling a small hand-held harp, the Celtic lyre we created has thirty-five strings and is suitable for concert or solo work as well as musical therapy and traditional folk music. John Billing, who plays the lyre all over the world, helped us to develop the instrument by advising us on sound and tone.'

The Celtic lyre project was made possible by a donation from the Arts Council for Northern Ireland Lottery Fund. 'Originally, it was supposed to be a one-year pilot scheme, running two days a week,' says Clifford. 'We put a lot of effort into it and the result was incredible. The culmination of the year's project was the performance in the Waterfront Hall, which sold out and which was attended by the Minister for Health, Bairbre de Brún, and Lady Hermon, MP for North Down as well as representatives from social services and the health and education boards. Afterwards, we were asked if we would play the National Concert Hall in Dublin, with the result that within twelve months we played the most prestigious venue in Belfast and the most prestigious venue in Dublin.'

It is important to Clifford that the Camphill residents – many of whom have mental, emotional and behavioural difficulties – are totally involved in the production process. The last few years have seen a gradual switch from the building of garden furniture to Celtic lyres, which are now in demand all over the world, with orders coming in from as far away as America and Japan. The emphasis, however, is on quality and careful craftsmanship rather than volume, with each instrument taking three months to complete. 'It is important to stress that from the initial selection of the timber to the final polishing process we use the individual skills of our special needs colleagues at Mourne Grange,' says Clifford, who runs the workshop with one other volunteer and a team of eight residents with intellectual disabilities. 'I believe that the qualities our residents bring to their work is reflected in the brightness and the warmth of tone of the instruments.

'We start with choosing the tree and preparing the wood: our lyres are constructed mainly from Irish hardwoods, especially elm and sycamore. We have an estate of some 150 acres at Mourne Grange, so we don't have any great difficulty in finding the right trees. We use European spruce for the soundboards and bracing and all our soundboards feature a unique bracing pattern, which is hand-carved and individually 'voiced'. Each person has a specific production task: four people use the machinery for cutting out the basic frames and everyone else is involved in gluing the frames together and in the whole finishing process.

'Our purpose is to provide an opportunity for special needs people to work on something highly creative at their own pace as well as producing musical instruments of great beauty, quality and individuality. For us, the real value of the instrument lies not in its financial worth, but in the great care that has gone into its production and the love that is involved in playing it. It is a very unusual project in that people are given the opportunity to be involved in the entire production process — from choosing the tree to playing the finished instrument. We are probably the only people in the world to have taken the lyre so far as to be actually performing with it in public and to have made CDs, while incorporating people with special needs into every single aspect of manufacture and performance.'

The orchestra has attracted widespread attention and performs regularly. 'We are in reasonable demand because our residents have a wonderful ability to perform,' says Clifford. 'People want us to come and play for them because the quality of the music is so high as well as the fact that it is an inclusive group, involving able-bodied people and people with disabilities. We can play with as little as three people or as many as one hundred, depending on the size of the venue.'

Clara Thomsen, who has lived at Mourne Grange for twenty-one years, did not find it difficult to learn to play the Celtic lyre. 'You just have to stroke it, like you would stroke an animal,' she says. 'You make the different notes by stroking the different strings: you mustn't pluck it, like a harp. When I have the music in front of me I have the letters written down, to help me, because the trouble is to know which notes to play.'

Some evenings Clara takes out her lyre and plays by herself for a while. Hilary Patterson, who has lived at Mourne Grange since it opened in 1971, also plays sometimes in the evenings. 'I find it relaxing to play,' she says. 'And when I go to bed I listen to a CD of lyre music to help me settle down. The doctor said I should listen to it at night because I was having problems sleeping.'

Hilary used to get very nervous before performing, but now she can't wait to get on stage. 'I was nervous the first couple of times – playing in front of a lot of people – but I've got used to it now,' she says. 'Seeing Mary McAleese after the concert in the National Concert Hall made me very nervous, though, because she is such an important person. Somebody took me by the hand and took me to talk to her. She said how nice the concert was and how well we had played. I was glad to get to meet her.'

Hilary's daily work in the community involves helping to look after an elderly lady as well as doing the ironing for three of the houses, each of which accommodates ten people. Clara, on the other hand, spends her time weaving headscarves. These are sold in the craft shop, which is open to the public five days a week. Both Clara and Hilary look forward to Thursday mornings when they join in rehearsals in the community's music room. These are led by John Billing and Anna Cooper, who is a music therapist based in Holywood, Co. Down. Once a month members of other Camphill communities (there are ten throughout Ireland, north and south) come to join in rehearsals.

Some members of the community are unable to read music or to play a melody and Clifford has made an instrument especially for them, thus ensuring that everyone who wants to play an instrument can. The polychord, which has ten strings, can be tuned to one specific chord or note – from A to G. Clifford has also built an 'in-between' instrument, the bodrún lyre, which goes from a simple note up to a chord. 'What makes the whole thing absolutely equal opportunity is that we have fifty or sixty special needs residents, all of whom are amateur musicians, playing alongside professional musicians,' says Clifford. 'From world-class musicians to people who can play only one note: it's very equal opportunity. Within two years of the project starting, our residents were playing on stage alongside the likes of Phil Coulter. He loved it and, on stage at the National Concert Hall, he told the audience, "I've played with the Boston Philharmonic Orchestra, I've played with the London Philharmonic Orchestra, but this beats it all." We accompanied him playing one of his songs — a beautiful piece called "Farewell to Inishowen".'

What do the residents get out of performing? 'Pride, privilege, dignity and equal opportunity, because they get the same opportunity as anybody else,' says Clifford. 'Some of their parents have said to me, "I would never have expected even my able-bodied son or daughter to achieve that." It's not just about building instruments and playing them; it's a very social project, with people travelling from all over Ireland and other parts of the world to play. It's about bringing people together to tune into each other in a different way — not conversing, but tuning in and listening to each other. Playing together is the most important thing.'

In May 2000 about twenty people from Camphill communities throughout Ireland attended the first ever international lyre conference in Hamburg, Germany, which was attended by some four hundred enthusiasts from all over the world. The Celtic lyre was widely admired by the other participants. In May 2003 they played at the Dumfries and Galloway Arts Festival in Scotland. The following month they performed at a Special Olympics symposium in Belfast City Hall and, in July, a twenty-strong contingent attended the second international lyre conference, which was held in New Hampshire, USA.

In 2002 Mourne Grange hosted a Celtic lyre summer school, which was attended by thirty people from overseas — including Germany, Switzerland, Japan and America. It was timed to coincide with a local folk festival and the orchestra performed at a number of local venues during the week. Clara, who is originally from Denmark, particularly enjoyed the week. 'I enjoyed people coming from other countries to stay,' she says. 'It's very joyful to get to know people from other countries: we got to know them and they got to know us. It was very nice.'

Clifford's background is neither in music or woodwork. For twenty years he was involved in his family's business of selling high-powered motorbikes – until his father had a stroke in 1980, which left him wheelchair-bound and unable to speak. Clifford spent the next fourteen years caring for him, during which time he came into contact with Camphill – an organisation started in Aberdeen in 1940 by a refugee from Vienna called Karl König. Now a world-wide movement, there are almost one hundred Camphill centres in twenty countries, working to create communities in which vulnerable children and adults can live, learn and work with others in healthy social relationships based on mutual care and respect.

The communities are based on the acceptance of the spiritual uniqueness of each human being, regardless of disability or religious or racial background. The insights of Rudolf Steiner provide the foundation for Camphill's work in curative education and community building, with the able-bodied and people with learning disabilities living, working and sharing together in a spirit of community where all members contribute what they can towards the well-being of their fellows.

In 1994 Clifford went to live at a Camphill community in Devon, in the south of England. After several years there he made plans to run a workshop in a community in America, but, with his father's health rapidly deteriorating, he decided against venturing so far, choosing to move to Ireland instead. 'My father was getting weaker and I couldn't bear to leave him,' says Clifford. 'He died three months after I came here, but I never moved on because this is just such a wonderful place to be! I felt at home the first time I set foot in Northern Ireland and I find the Mournes particularly beautiful. I ride my bike first thing every morning and head up into the hills, where there is a great beauty and a stark cleanliness. When you live and work amid such beauty it helps the creative process.'

What attracted Clifford to Camphill in the first place? 'Just the peacefulness and the way that there is a dignity and an absolute equanimity in the realm between carer and handicapped person. We are subtly different from most other organisations in that everybody who works here is a volunteer – nobody receives a salary. We pool all the money and we live in a community. We all get our board and lodging, but we believe very much that because all our residents are working to keep the community running in the same way as us, then why should we get paid if they don't? They may be doing different kind of work than us, but that work keeps the community functioning. Without them, the community wouldn't function.

'The spiritual life of the community is another big attraction: we have a very strong spiritual base, which is non-denominational. It's a Christian base and we're working towards peace between human beings. Other benefits of community life include mutual understanding and support. We share everything with the special needs residents – their highs and their lows – and they share ours. It's like living in an extended family – not in a New Age kind of way, but a real living together as a community. We share each other's lives in a deep way – the good and the bad.'

Has day-to-day living with people with special needs changed Clifford in any way? 'Yes. Every day one is reminded of one's own failings and inability to meet the world in an open and honest way. People with learning disabilities are so free and connected to the world. Living and working together allows mutual understanding, trust and support to exist between carer and cared for.'

While a part of him continues to hanker to go to America, Clifford is in no doubt that his future lies with Camphill in Ireland. 'Apart from anything else, the Celtic lyre project is too good to leave: it encompasses not only all of my ideals, but all of my energy as well. It is remarkable that the people involved – Sam, John and myself – have come together unexpectedly in the way that we have. It is almost as if the Celtic lyre project was an idea whose time had come. I'm very much a down-to-earth person, but, believe me, this is sheer magic! There is no other way to describe it.'

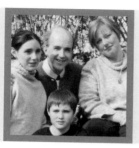

Lorraine Leake

*... who believes the health services have a
greater role to play in supporting families*

IT IS A COMMON SIGHT, DURING competitions at the music college in
Cork, to see a lady in a wheelchair at the bottom of the stairs, listening
intently to any snatches of music that drift down from the hall where the
competitors are in performance.

The lady in question is Lorraine Leake, who was diagnosed with
multiple sclerosis (MS) when she was twenty-four and who has used a
wheelchair since 1996. She enjoys listening to her thirteen-year-old
daughter, Angela, practising at home on the piano, violin and flute and,
like any proud mother, loves to support her during competitions.
Unfortunately, however, the lack of wheelchair facilities in the college
means that she has no way of actually seeing her daughter perform. All
she can do is listen at the bottom of the stairs.

Usually someone thinks to run down to her and say, 'Angela's playing
now', although this is completely unnecessary. Lorraine always knows
when her daughter is performing: after all, she hears her practising every

single day at home. Despite the fact that she cannot make it into the hall, Lorraine will always insist on attending her daughter's competitions. 'It can be very painful for her, and for me, knowing that I can't see her perform in public, but I want her to know that I support her and I'm there for her,' says Lorraine. 'I know I'm in a wheelchair and that it's not always possible to make all of society wheelchair-friendly, but I want to support her in any way that I can.'

Angela was six years old when her mother first used a wheelchair; her brother, Joseph, was five. Lorraine is painfully aware that at times this has been 'really awful' for them. While she can drive her kids around in her specially adapted car, she needs their help getting in and out because she simply has not the strength to do it on her own. And, while they are more or less used to this now, the children have both been through stages of acute embarrassment.

'I remember one time, a few years ago, when I arrived home with Joseph and one of his friends was in the driveway with his mother. Joseph said to me, "Oh please, Mummy, don't get out of the car; I'll be so embarrassed. Please don't do it." I told him I had to because he was going out with his friend and, if he didn't help me out, I'd be stuck in the car for three hours until his dad came home. It's so hard because I have needs, but I do respect where they are coming from as well.'

Lorraine regrets the fact that her children's lives have been severely restricted as a result of her condition. 'While I have come to terms with having MS, I don't like it because it's putting huge restrictions not only on my life, but also on my husband's and children's lives. My husband, Joe, and my children have supported me so much over the years; they've been my primary carers. When my husband goes out to work, my children have to help me a lot, which curtails their fun. Every time we go out as a family, they have to think, "Can we bring Mammy there? Will there be a ramp? Will there be facilities for her to use the bathroom?" MS has not only encroached on my life, but also on theirs. The most crushing thing of all was when my husband said to me recently, "You know, Lorraine, I have known you much longer with MS than I have without." It's the same with the children: they've only ever known me dependent on them. It is awful for them.'

It is hardly the kind of family life that Lorraine and Joe had imagined when they married in 1989 and moved into their dream house in the Cork suburb of Douglas. The dream started to disintegrate after the birth of Joseph when Lorraine found herself becoming unsteady on her feet. Whereas, during the pregnancy, she had been walking eight miles a day, with Angela in the buggy, now she could hardly walk around her garden without falling over. 'I went all of a sudden from being a great walker to being confined to the house. And that was an awful shock. I had been so active, but my co-ordination was gradually getting worse and I had to start using a stick. A couple of years later I started to use a rollator – a frame on wheels.'

Joe made a special path so that Lorraine could walk down the garden to see their fruit and vegetables. They were trying to be as self-sufficient as possible, including making their own preserves. But a time came when it was no longer possible for Lorraine to use the special path and the only way she could manage the stairs in the house was by bumping down on her behind. 'We had no downstairs toilet and every time I had to go upstairs I felt like I was climbing Mount Everest,' remembers Lorraine.

It was at this point, four years after moving into their dream home, that the Leakes reluctantly decided there was nothing for it but to sell up and move into a bungalow. By this time Lorraine had received a diagnosis of MS, which she knew to be a progressive condition. 'I'll always remember the day I opened the envelope and saw the words "multiple sclerosis". I went into shock – complete shock. I didn't sleep at all that night; I was shivering and shaking all night long. I had known somebody who had MS and it seemed awful: when you've known somebody when they were well and then you see them in a wheelchair, you draw many fearful conclusions.

'I'd say I've been through all the emotions over the years and I am probably still going through them – anger, frustration, sadness and grief. Sadness and grief are the biggest ones – grief for something I've lost because I had always thoroughly enjoyed walking and appreciated every minute of it, so it's really hard to know why that was taken off me. I often ask, "Why me?", but I think that's normal. It's so sad that I can't go for a walk now with my husband; we have a lovely garden and I can't even play in it with my children. They can bring me down the garden, but when they're helping me we change roles: they become adult-children because they are my hands and legs.

'Sometimes I feel like I'm a parasite and they're the host because I constantly need them. I always seem to be saying, "Could you get me this or that?" I seem to spend the day calling out for help and it's hard on those around me because it must seem like, "Jeepers, she always needs something". I can't even go to the wardrobe and take out clothes for myself and I can't do much in the kitchen; at this stage I mainly supervise and tell the others what needs to be done. My co-ordination isn't great at the moment and I need meat to be chopped up for me, so just when we've sat down to a nice meal, "your one over there is wanting hers chopped up again".

'Not only do my children have to cook, but they also have to help me sit up, get dressed, get me into the wheelchair and help me in the bathroom. And, in the afternoons when I'm too tired to push myself in the wheelchair, they have to push me from one room to another. It is so frustrating for me and for my family. My life is higgledy-piggledy and I really need as much help to try and make my way through life. I have as much a right to a life as anybody else. All the relationships have changed within the family and it's not right. They are my support system – they do what I ask – but there are times they would like not to do it. They do it because they love their mother, but they've no support.

'It has been my experience that when one person in a couple is seriously ill the healthy spouse is expected to give up work to mind their partner. That seems very unjust to deny one person their right to work when some home help could mean that the healthy spouse can continue to go out to work and get a break from the vicious cycle. Society in general, and the health board in particular, expects the family to care for the person with MS. Yet it is no longer expected that women stay at home to mind their children, so don't you think it's discrimination to expect more from the couple visited by illness? I didn't bring on my illness – nor did my family – so why is it we are being plunged into taking full responsibility for it?'

Lorraine feels strongly that the role of primary carer should not fall on the family. 'Those in authority feel that families must help out, but I don't believe they should be the primary carers. It is compulsory altruism – they have to give all the time – but they have no support. Absolutely none. Who helps them when they get frustrated and angry? My children have been robbed of so much – they really have – and there's no support for them. There have been times when they've become angry and frustrated, and obviously that's a natural feeling because they're having to do something they really don't want to do, but who do they talk to?

'It might be right for them to feel angry, but getting angry with their mother isn't always right because, although I have MS, I am not MS. There is a difference. I am a person first, trying to live my life fully; and my husband and children help me to live as fully as I can. I've explained to the children why I need so much help – that it's not my choice – MS comes part and parcel with me, unfortunately, and I need the help because there's no support services there. I do understand their frustration and anger, but it's very hard when they get angry. Until recently they confused MS with their mother, but mother is not MS: I am a person first and, unfortunately, I have to drag this MS around with me. Now, as they get older, they're beginning to see the difference.'

When the children were small the Leakes employed an au pair, but after a few years they found this was no longer financially viable. Instead, they opted for a home help to assist with domestic duties three hours a day, freeing up Lorraine to spend time with Angela and Joseph. 'That's my role as a mother,' she says. 'I've always done loads of things with them: we read together and we watch videos. When they were smaller, I used to love reading them Roald Dahl books.'

In November 2002, however, the home help left and the Southern Health Board could not find a replacement. For six weeks the only outside help Lorraine received was a visit from a nurse once a week to help her in the bathroom. 'I need to use the toilet more than once a week, so obviously my husband and children were doing the other times,' she says. 'When the children came home from school they had to help cook and clean and then put Mummy to bed. Over the Christmas period my daughter was doing all the shopping and the housework, which I felt was scandalous.'

Three months after the home help left, Lorraine put pen to paper and wrote a letter to *The Irish Examiner* in which she detailed her circumstances. 'I decided to stand up for myself because I had all this frustration inside me, which I couldn't take any longer. I was getting no support and I felt I was exploiting my husband and children. I just wrote the plain truth – that my children had been helping me for seven years and I didn't think they should be my primary carers. All I was asking was that the health services would share the load. That's all I've been asking for years.'

The letter paid off because, within a fortnight, the health board gave the go ahead for Lorraine to get a personal assistant from the Cork Centre for Independent Living. 'I had been waiting for months to hear if they would sanction a PA. My husband and children had been carrying the load, but they don't get paid for those duties. Personally, I feel they should be given honorary nursing degrees because they've gone beyond the call of duty. When something goes wrong, they've nobody to ask advice from. They've had no training and there is no back up; they have nobody to ring and talk to when they get frustrated. That is not good enough.'

Life in the Leake household has been transformed for the ten hours a week that PA, Sinéad O'Riordain, is around. Her primary role is to assist Lorraine with personal care. 'It's made a huge difference because it means, for ten hours a week, my husband and my children are not responsible for me. The children want to see their mother and my husband wants to see his wife, but often when they interact with me it's duty that comes first: they're playing the role of carer. Pushing your mother into the bathroom and stripping her down: they have seen their mum at her most vulnerable. It's been very hard for them. Having said that, we are also the best of friends. Now my family has ten hours a week that they do not have to undertake personal care duties, so I am no longer asking them to help me *all* the time.'

In 2001 Lorraine completed a course in disability studies at University College Cork. She found it somewhat 'depressing', but at least it gave her the confidence to challenge the state services. One time when her hours of physiotherapy were unexpectedly cut, she fought to be given equipment at home. 'I insisted that, if physiotherapy wasn't going to be provided for me, which I was eager to get, then I ought to get equipment I could use at home. In the end the health board provided a motomed – an electric bicycle for wheelchair users – and I can do three kilometres a day on it, for which I'm ever so grateful. I also got a standing frame, but I had to fight really, really hard – I mean I was vicious. I had to push for years: I just kept repeating myself, like a broken record, saying that I wanted to exercise in order to keep as much mobility as possible. I wrote letters, using language I had picked up from the course. But fighting takes a lot of energy and I don't have much energy; when I fight it whacks me for other duties, like looking after my family.'

Lorraine found it 'scandalous' that the Irish government planned to purchase two brand new aeroplanes for the Taoiseach in 2003 at a time when there were widespread cutbacks in the health service. 'The money could have provided home help and personal assistance for those in society struggling to survive. I have lived with MS for twelve years and

I am constantly frustrated by the exclusion imposed by society on people with disabilities. I get offered Prozac for my difficulties; the Taoiseach gets two state of the art jets. It doesn't seem very just. How quickly state money — which is my money, too — can be used to buy aeroplanes because the poor Taoiseach is frustrated. When I'm frustrated with the footpaths, or whatever, it's presumed I need Prozac, whereas what's needed is a change within society to include the person with disabilities. Prozac really isn't the answer; it's not a long term solution.'

Once a week Lorraine attends the Practical School of Philosophy in Cork where she practises meditation. She also listens to relaxing music and meditates at home for twenty minutes every day, which helps alleviate tension. It was suggested from a number of quarters that smoking cannabis might help her relax, but she reckoned 'blotting out reality' would only cause more problems and would not allow her to fully participate in life.

'I did weigh up the choice and contemplated whether cannabis would actually make my MS better and I decided that, really, what I am looking for is something to take the bloody MS away. That's what I'm really looking for. When you're ill you will do anything to get better because you feel desperate. I would eat wallpaper — I really would — if I thought it would make me better. I'd love to be well enough to go out and work, but I'm denied that because of this awful disease.'

Since her diagnosis, Lorraine has done much 'soul-searching', which has resulted in a changed attitude towards life. 'Now I think it's better just to live each day as it comes because there is no point in worrying about tomorrow. I have learned to enjoy the simple things — I love reading and I enjoy looking at my plants. I have a gorgeous camellia outside my living room window and I'm so lucky that I can see its colours and textures. And I'm lucky I can hear my children play their music.'

Lorraine can only hope, as time goes by, that she will get more and more support from the wider community, thereby freeing her family to pursue their own interests. 'Please God, my children will go to college because I don't want them exploited any more,' she says. 'I don't want their lives locked up in MS and caring all the time. I feel they've done their bit. Now it's time to leave them alone.'

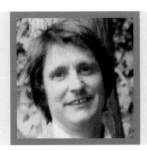

Ivan Pratt

... a businessman who describes reading as like
driving with the handbrake on

'YOU KNOW, I WAS DOING REALLY BADLY IN SCHOOL and so I went to get checked out to see if I had dyslexia. But it turned out I was just really thick!'

Ivan Pratt roared laughing when he heard a stand-up comedian tell this joke on television a few years ago. As a dyslexic of high intelligence, he had good reason to enjoy this particular wisecrack. Ivan's schooldays had been a struggle, but he had always known he was not 'thick': an IQ test at the age of four had proved it.

His parents, Donald and Hilary Pratt, who founded the successful Avoca Handweavers chain in 1974, took a fairly laid back approach to Ivan's education. Knowing that he was a smart kid, but that he found it a struggle to demonstrate his knowledge on paper, they did not have high academic expectations of him. 'It won't matter after school; life is more important,' his father used to tell him. Once he finished fifth year of secondary school, Ivan's parents told him he could leave school, if he wished. He was thrilled with their suggestion and seized the opportunity to drive the Avoca van. Twenty years on, he is now a director of the family business.

Not only were his parents understanding, but his teachers were, too. They knew that a lot of information was 'going in', even if it was far from obvious from his essays and exam scripts. For, as a dyslexic, Ivan struggled with reading and writing (the word 'dyslexia' comes from Greek and literally means 'difficulty with words'). On top of his difficulties with literacy, he could not grasp much beyond the basics of mathematics (he used to confuse the numbers eleven and twelve – a common dyslexic trait) and he could never remember his left from his right. Problems with numeracy and directions are common characteristics of dyslexia, too. In the end, he did manage to master his left and right by remembering it was his right thumb that he sucked!

Although people with dyslexia can make great progress, it is not a condition that can be simply shaken off. After all, the 'wiring' in the brain cannot be altered (dyslexia is thought to be caused by the right hemisphere of the brain interfering with the sequential processing of verbal stimuli, which occurs in the left hemisphere). Even now, Ivan finds that reading is 'like driving with the handbrake on; it just drags.'

He believes he was fortunate that his dyslexia was picked up fairly early on. His first teacher at St Patrick's National School, Dalkey, south Dublin, believed that 'nothing was going in'. Fearing she had a 'retarded' child on her hands, Hilary took her four-year-old son to a psychiatrist who diagnosed 'cross-laterality'. Three years later she took him to a University of Wales dyslexic centre in Bangor, Wales where, after a full day of tests, she was told they had never before come across anyone 'so dyslexic'. Her son would need twenty times more teaching than a non-dyslexic child to reach the same level. They did say, however, that Ivan was 'smart enough – there's nothing wrong with his intelligence – although he does have a learning disability.'

A short time later Ivan moved to Brook House where his mother took him out of class during Irish lessons to help him with his reading and writing, until the school appointed a remedial teacher. For his secondary education, Ivan was enrolled into Sandford Park, Ranelagh where, again, instead of learning languages, a special-needs teacher helped him with literacy. 'That gave me good enough English, although my spelling's not great,' says Ivan. 'I used to always confuse "b" and "d" until my sister, Amanda, told me that if you write the word 'bed' it looks like a bed; that helped me remember and I learned to do it automatically in my head. I still use this rule. I know my silent "k"s, like knife and knowledge, and I can always remember to spell "right" without any problem, but other spellings didn't go in and I'd make the same error time and time again. I've no idea why.'

To this day, Ivan hates his handwriting; he is very self-conscious about it. 'I only write for myself – things like appointments in my diary,' he says. 'I don't even like leaving my diary open in my office in case other people see my writing, although I can write reasonably well, if I make the effort. I don't write any Christmas cards and my poor wife, Caroline, knows when I write her a card it almost kills me. And, although I take telephone messages, I never write them down. There's ways around most things and, when I'm writing emails, I use the spell check and, if I have to send an official letter, then I'll get someone to type it for me. When I write a cheque or a letter I always get somebody to check it, although it drives me absolutely mad when they point out a mistake. I can see the fault as soon as they point it out, which is absolutely infuriating. Cheques are used so seldom now, thank goodness – it's all Laser and Visa. It used to be that when I walked into a shop I would have a quick look at the sign outside before going in, to see how to spell the name of the shop, in case I wanted to buy something.'

Ivan's parents have always encouraged him to be open with people about his dyslexia and those he works closely with at Kilmacanogue, Co. Wicklow all know of his condition. 'The people I work with are fantastic,' he says. 'It can be terribly irritating for everybody else – if I ask how to spell a particular word and twenty minutes later I go back to write the same word and I have to ask again because I can't remember how to spell it. Every now and again someone who knows I have dyslexia will ask me how to spell something and I reply that if I learned how to spell that I would probably forget how to spell Ivan! Some spellings stay in my head but, for some reason, others just don't stick. I don't know why.'

When he was in school, Ivan's classmates knew about his struggles with reading and writing, despite his best efforts to cover up his page while he was writing. He was never teased or bullied, however, and he was always popular. 'I never remember feeling stupid because my dyslexia was identified and understood by my teachers and parents at such a young age,' says Ivan. 'I found I could relate to people at the bottom of the class and the top of the class and I was never picked on. I became one of the jokers of the class: I always had a smart comment to make to prove that I was not an idiot.'

Ivan did not put himself under too much pressure over his studies until his mock Intermediate Certificate exams loomed on the horizon. 'I did try and study in the evenings, but I found it so tiring,' he says. 'I became a nervous wreck for months and months, but I think a huge amount of people did, anyway. It was such fear because I knew I was so far behind.'

Two years before he was due to take his first state exam Hilary had requested the Department of Education to allow Ivan to be assessed by dictaphone, rather than by writing (she had heard of another student who had been allowed to do this). She 'fought and fought' until, finally, with only one week to go before the exams were due to start, Ivan was given the go ahead. In a sense, however, it was too little too late. 'It's hard to speak an essay onto tape and there was no time for me to have any training to do that,' he says.

'I got to the point that the fear was so much that I just didn't care anymore. I had cared about the mocks so much – I was terrified doing them and I didn't sleep for a week beforehand – but, by the time it came to the actual Inter, I had gone beyond caring. Maybe because life had continued as normal after the mock, I realised the same would happen after the Inter. In the end I got better results writing in the mock than I did with a tape recorder in the real thing. It was so cringe-worthy getting my results. It always was, the whole way through my educational career, and I am sure all people with learning difficulties feel the same. If you feel you're relatively intelligent, to get the kind of results I did is sickening. I've always felt our education system shouldn't be geared totally towards reading and writing; I think it's unfair that some people are not allowed to blossom until after they leave school. I didn't feel this for me – as I am not arty, musical or sporty – but for those who are it seems a little unfair.'

Ivan's passion during his teenage years was the drums and he attended weekly lessons in Dalkey. 'I was appalling at it, but I was enthusiastic,' he says, with characteristic modesty. 'My drumming teacher told me one day, "Ivan, people tell you that your schooldays are the best years of your life. Don't believe that for one second – they're the worst." And it's true – although my schooldays weren't particularly bad, they certainly weren't the best.'

Ivan did not give a second's thought to his answer when his parents asked him if he would like to leave school at the end of fifth year. He was thrilled at the prospect of liberation from the classroom. He had a great time over the summer, but it was a different story when all his friends returned to school in September. 'I was delighted at first and I loved driving the company van, but I soon lost touch with everybody,' he says. 'I felt I'd burnt my bridges and that, maybe, I should have stuck at school. I had no choice but to work for the family company. Who else would have me?'

Three years later, Ivan was feeling 'miserable' and thinking he would like to 'do something' for himself when his father suggested he refurbish a warehouse he owned on Lotts Lane (behind Bachelors Walk), but had been unable to let for some time. Ivan and a mate spent the next year doing up the premises with the intention of turning it into a music studio and, shortly before the work was complete, their first customers walked in the door. 'I had just climbed down the ladder so I could turn up the radio because The Waterboys' song 'The Whole of the Moon' (which was number two in the British charts at the time) had just come on,' remembers Ivan. 'I heard voices behind me and turned around to find The Waterboys standing right behind us! We hadn't heard them come in and they'd already wandered around the premises. They asked how soon they could have a room and we told them straightaway. They used the studios as their base for the next five years.'

Ivan was thrilled to have something that he could really throw himself into. He spent all day every day at the studios — even on a Sunday morning, his parents would hear the click of the front door at seven o'clock as Ivan set off into town. Some nights he even slept in the studios. 'Over the years we had some really big acts in and one time Howard Jones had millions of pounds worth of computer equipment there. Our insurance would never have covered it and my partner and I decided to take turns sleeping in the studios because we were afraid of the equipment being stolen. It was such a great break we didn't tell Howard Jones' management we weren't insured to cover that amount of equipment!'

The experience of running the studios completely changed Ivan. 'I adored running it because it was mine and, for the first time in my life, I had responsibility. It totally changed me as a person. But, after about five years, I realised I didn't want to work in the music business long-term because it wasn't structured enough as a career. About that time my father was made an offer for the building, which gave me an honourable way out of the business.'

Ivan returned to the family firm where he became involved in the manufacturing and wholesale side of the business. He returned a different person than when he first started at seventeen and he soon came to enjoy his work. 'I was very lucky to be able to work for the family business because, if I'd been born in not so lucky circumstances, my only way of getting ahead would have been through great exam results. I remember my parents asked me, when I was about twelve, what I wanted to do when I left school. I was really into aeroplanes at the time and I said I wanted to be a pilot. They said, 'Listen, you're never going to get the exams to be a pilot'.

'I knew I was never going to get anywhere through academia, but I never had to because the family business was always there. And it doesn't matter now because I adore my work – I eat, sleep and drink it. Dyslexia has been an inconvenience, but I've learned to live with it. It's frustrating at times, but I think all people have inconveniences. Everyone around me has always known I have dyslexia. All my teachers knew and, in fact, they let me away with murder because of it.'

Ivan is convinced that he would be a very different person if he had not experienced problems with literacy. 'Dyslexia definitely shaped me because you spend so much of your childhood in school and I think it's obvious that anything that plays such a part in your childhood will shape you as a person,' he says. 'Because I struggled in school I understand people better. I think having dyslexia has made me very good at working with people: I'm relatively good at showing people how to do things because, for so many years, people were showing me what to do. I think it's made me a much more understanding person and a softer person because I wasn't always swimming along at the top of the class.'

As a child, Monday mornings used to fill Ivan with dread. In fact, he was affected so deeply that, to this day, he still experiences anxiety at the start of each week. 'Friday was always such a relief, when school was over for the week,' he remembers, 'But then the anxiety would build up during Sunday for the dreaded Monday morning. I still get that anxiety and so I come into work for a few hours every Sunday to ease myself slowly into the week's work. I find it much easier on a Monday morning if I've checked my emails and done other jobs the day before. It may seem stupid, but it works for me.'

In some respects, even though his education was such a struggle, Ivan regrets that he did not pursue his studies further. 'I felt pretty bad, actually, when I left school,' he says. 'I felt like I was copping out by taking the easy way out. When I was a teenager sitting in a classroom, listening to a teacher going on about some aspect of history or geography, I wasn't really very interested. But I'd love it now if somebody told me about all those things; and if they read Shakespeare to me. I wouldn't go back to education now, though, because I love what I do and we feel we have a lot more to achieve with Avoca. It would probably be good for me to do an Irish Management Institute course, but I would be worried to do it because there would be far too much reading and arithmetic and I don't know how it would go.

'I wish reading wasn't such a chore for me. I can read, but it just doesn't flow very easily. I love listening to interesting programmes on the radio because the information just flows out. I'll pick up *The Irish Times* and read the bits that interest me, but I would love to read far more books and I always have a few lined up. However, when I pick up a book I choose it carefully because, as far as I'm concerned, if I'm going to spend most of my holidays reading it I don't want to get halfway through only to discover it's rubbish. I love bringing a good book on holidays and, once I get into one, I bore everyone about it. I usually read factual books – often books about family businesses, similar to Avoca – maybe just to get inspiration or ideas. In saying that, I did enjoy Nick Hornby's last few books.'

Dyslexia is thought to be genetic, although no-one else in the Pratt family is affected by it. If Ivan had a child with dyslexia, how would he help him or her? 'I wouldn't do anything any different than the way it was done for me,' he says. 'I'd tell them not to worry about it – not to get too caught up in it – but to try the best they can. I would say to anybody with a learning disability, 'Don't sit there struggling with a form, with beads of sweat coming off you – say you'll bring it back later. Take it away and ask somebody to help you – somebody you're not embarrassed to ask. I never ask a stranger; I always prefer to ask a member of my family.'

Looking back, Ivan feels he has led 'a charmed life'. He says, 'I'm lucky that I was able to go into the family business and I'm lucky that my family and teachers put a huge amount of energy into getting my reading and writing up to a level where I can read and write to a reasonable standard. However, I am very dyslexic and most people who are affected by dyslexia do not need as much time as I did to get on top of reading and writing.

'At the end of the day, dyslexia can't be that bad,' he adds. 'After all, Einstein had it. And you can't get any better than that!'

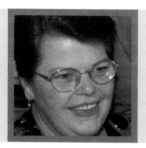

Ann Pepper

... a wheelchair user who volunteers at the local resource centre

ANN PEPPER CAN JUST ABOUT REMEMBER the last time she set foot upstairs in her house. It was four years ago. The experience was such a nightmare she vowed never to attempt it again.

'I crawled up the stairs and it took too much out of me,' recalls Ann, 'After I bumped back down, I said to myself, "I can't do this anymore, I can't".'

Not that she would not love to go up the stairs of her Tallaght home and give the place a good spring clean. She dare not even begin to imagine what state the place is in, what with her two youngest offspring, twenty-three year old Gareth and fourteen-year-old Dean, still living at home. From time to time she asks them to bring down the towels to be washed and the rubbish bin to be emptied and daughter Linda – who lives in nearby Killinarden estate – often checks upstairs during her frequent visits to the house.

The downstairs, however, is Ann's pride and joy. As well as dusting and hoovering, she does all the cooking, washing and ironing. 'I hate to see things not done in the house and I think that's what keeps me going,' she says. 'I muddle through. I have a disability — it doesn't have me, and it won't get me. I'm a fighter and I'm not going to give up.'

Linda's four-year-old grandson, Jordan, helps keep her spirits up. 'I call him "my little sunshine" because he's the light of my heart. One day he asked me why I called him that and I told him, "It's because, when you're around, you light me up." Being a granny is great! You do things differently with your grandchildren: you get a second chance at everything and you enjoy it more,' says Ann, who has six children and five grandchildren.

They all got a terrible shock the day Ann arrived home in a wheelchair. 'I had gone into Beaumont Hospital that morning walking, but barely walking: I was wearing a splint on my right leg and there was a dreadful infection in it. It was very painful and I was in a bad way. When an occupational therapist said I would be taken into hospital, I told her, 'Look, I can't be taken in because I've too much to do — I've a family to look after.' The neurologist, Dr Orla Hardiman, said I could return home that day, but that it would have to be in a wheelchair. I had never imagined I would end up in a wheelchair. It was a great disappointment.'

Ann had been feeling unwell for several years — from the time she started nursing her partner after he was diagnosed with cancer in 1996. Any tiredness, headaches, aches and pains she experienced at that time she put down to the inevitable exhaustion that came from being a full-time carer. She never thought there was anything wrong, even though she suffered 'dreadful, dreadful' pain in her back while walking.

One day, while accompanying her partner to an appointment at Beaumont Hospital, a poster on the wall caught her eye. It simply said, 'What happens after polio?' The word 'polio' rang a bell with Ann because, as a child, she had had polio and, from the age of four to thirteen, had lived in a rehabilitation centre run by the Central Remedial Clinic (CRC). 'I took down the contact number, stuck it in my handbag and completely forgot about it,' she says.

Following the death of her partner, which came nineteen weeks after diagnosis, Ann was surprised to find her health continuing to deteriorate. After a particularly bad fall down the stairs, which resulted in a sprained wrist, multiple bruising and a horrific mark on the side of her face (where she hit a cupboard in the hall), she decided it was time to seek help. 'I just couldn't take any more of it, so I went to see my GP. He thought it could have been to do with '"the change of life". I said to him, "You don't fall down the stairs with the mid-life" I didn't go back to him.'

Some months later Ann was rooting through her bag when she came across the number she had scribbled on a scrap of paper at Beaumont Hospital. When she plucked up the courage to ring the number, she found herself talking to Joan Bradley, secretary of the Post Polio Support Group. A polio survivor herself, Joan proceeded to ask Ann a number of questions.

'She asked if I ever got tired and I said, "Yes, once it gets to the afternoon I'm whacked." She asked if I was losing power in the leg that had been affected by polio. I was. As I answered her questions it became clear that I had all the classic symptoms of post-polio syndrome (PPS), which, until then, was something I had never heard of. She sent me a booklet about the condition and, when I read it, I felt I was reading all about me because I had every single symptom. So I went to my GP, got a referral letter and that's how I ended up in Beaumont.

'Dr Hardiman and Joan Bradley saved my sanity because, with the headaches, I thought I had a brain tumour — that's what runs in my family. I was sure I had one and I thought the doctors were stupid that they couldn't see that. I would wake up with a headache and I would go to bed with a headache; it turns out that is one of the symptoms of PPS.'

Up to 50 per cent of people who have polio as a child go on to develop PPS. This usually occurs between ten and forty years after they have recovered from the initial attack of the poliomyelitis virus. Symptoms include fatigue, slowly progressive muscle weakness and, at times, muscular atrophy.

Ann cannot remember when she was first affected by polio — she was only three years old at the time. She does, however, remember being brought to the CRC when she was four. Left sitting outside the doctor's door, she could clearly hear her mother telling the doctor that she 'needed a break'. At the time Ann had no idea what that meant — it wasn't until she was an adult that she realised her mother had meant a break from her. The doctor called Ann into the room and asked her if she would like to go on holiday with lots of other girls and boys. Of course, she said she would. She had no idea the 'holiday' meant going into hospital.

Despite such a deceptive introduction to rehabilitation and the fact that her right leg was severely affected by polio (she wore a calliper), Ann has many positive memories of her childhood years. 'They were good years because the staff were very good to me,' she recalls.

Her principle regret is how little education she received. 'I realise now that I didn't have a proper education. Rehab involved physiotherapy and a little schooling, but not a great deal. A retired teacher used to come in for a while each day, but it wasn't enough.'

Ann returned to her Finglas home on her confirmation day and, when she turned fifteen, started to attend a CRC workshop where she learned to use a sewing machine. A year later she took her first job — stitching the inside seam of ladies' garments in a clothing factory in Gardiner Street. The day she turned eighteen she moved out of home into a rented flat. Having spent so many years away from home, she had found it impossible to settle into a home environment: she barely knew her younger siblings and secretly longed for the day she could move out of home.

'I did all the things everybody does: I grew up and worked and, when I was twenty, I got married, had a family and ran a home,' says Ann. 'I had never heard of PPS, but I wish that somebody had warned me about it because, if I'd known polio could have put me in a wheelchair, I would have done things very differently. For a start, I wouldn't have had six children because I didn't bring my children into the world to look after me. That's the truth. I'm their Mammy and I'm the one who looks after them. I love my children and I love my grandchildren, but there's times I push myself too far; I'd literally be so exhausted that I wouldn't sleep for nights on end. Now it's not every polio survivor that gets PPS – it's usually brought on by surgery or stress. In my case, it was the stress of looking after my partner when he was ill.'

When Ann first arrived home in a wheelchair, she felt so miserable she 'just sat in a corner', with the result that the household chores fell on Linda, who at that time was still living at home. 'She had to take over until I adapted myself. She did all the washing, cooking and cleaning until, one day, she wasn't there and I took off one footrest on the wheelchair and, using my good leg, I learned to scoot around. That's the way I go around at home now and I do all my washing, drying, ironing and cooking and I do all the cleaning downstairs.'

For several years Anne was forced to sleep on the couch – until, that is, South Dublin County Council built an extension onto her house. 'I could have had a new bedroom and bathroom built on, but I didn't want my bedroom too far away from the family, so they turned my old kitchen into a bedroom and they built on a lovely new kitchen, utility room and bathroom. I had to wait a couple of years for that to be done.

'You do learn that you have to adapt. I have adapted because I have had no choice, but I'd love to be walking again. If I was to be granted one wish it would be to walk again. I wouldn't be looking to walk without a limp – just to be able to walk and to do the things I used to be able to do, like gardening. I had a beautiful garden before I went into a wheelchair; now it's just grass.

'I remember being on a course one day and a woman – an able-bodied woman – talked about how it was a great struggle for her every morning organising her children to go out to school, getting their breakfast, opening the curtains and putting out the bin. I was sitting there, just listening, and when it came to my turn to say something I said, "Ladies, you don't know how lucky you are. I'd love to be able to do all them things – open the curtains, run up and down the stairs, put out the bins and walk the children to school. You are so lucky that you are able to do those things. That's a gift". 'They were dumbfounded and there was total silence in the room. I said, "Now, I didn't mean to upset anybody, but we all have our gifts. Every time you're struggling putting out your bin, think how lucky you are that you're able to put it out. Or to be able to walk in the snow. Or even to walk in the rain." I have rain gear, but I hate wearing it. It looks horrible and I hate putting it on. *I hate it!* I'd rather get wet. People always say to me, "You're soaking", and I reply, "Isn't it great to be alive to know that you're wet?"'

The course Ann was attending was one of many on which she has enrolled at Killinarden Resource Centre. In fact, there isn't a single course at the centre in which she has not participated. Consumer awareness, aromatherapy, floristry, cookery, women's health, oil painting, knitting and crocheting, personal development, active and concerned citizens and parenting – she has a certificate for each and every one. The centre, which she first attended seven years ago, has proved a lifeline, even though she was 'petrified' when she signed up for her first course - personal development. 'It did me the power of good, though, because I learned loads about myself and, by the end, I was saying to myself, "Right, that's it. This is my life now and I'm grabbing hold of it." When I finished the course I went into counselling; I have always had a lot of confidence, but I wear a lot of masks as well. I still go to a counselling session every Monday afternoon and, for that hour, I wear no mask at all. And it's great not to wear one.'

Ann finds the sessions useful for exploring her feelings about being in a wheelchair. 'It was a huge kick in the behind to come home that day in a wheelchair. It really, really was. And no matter how much I was told that going into a wheelchair was not about giving up, but a part of saving and preserving what I had, I just didn't see it that way. All I could see was that I couldn't walk and so I started staying at home. I wouldn't go out because I didn't want anybody to see me in a wheelchair. I didn't want to give into the fact that this was me now for the rest of my life. But I realise now that if it wasn't for the wheelchair I wouldn't be able to go to the resource centre. I would be stuck at home looking at the soaps, listening to the radio and being depressed.

'I haven't come to terms with my disability and I know I will never get used to being in a wheelchair. At the end of the day, it's a huge thing to be stuck in a wheelchair because you can't possibly do the things you used to be able to do. There is pain with PPS – some days it is very little, other days it is greater – but I just adapt. The days I'm in a lot of pain, I still get out of bed and keep a routine. If I said to myself, "I won't go out today", then I know I wouldn't go out the next day either. I just do as much as I can and, if something's not done, it's not done. So what? The delph isn't shouting at me from the sink, "Wash me", and the ironing isn't saying, "Please run an iron over me". I have my good days and bad days, just like anybody else.'

Ann has become an invaluable helper at the resource centre, welcoming new people, making tea and coffee and, when the receptionists are taking their breaks, answering the telephones and taking the names of people as they arrive to attend courses. For eighteen months she helped in the creche, but it got 'too much' for her. However, she still helps organise Christmas parties for the children as well as for the over-55s who attend the 'Young at Heart' friendship group. In recognition of her tireless voluntary work, RTÉ's Joe Duffy presented her with an award at a special reception held in the centre in February 2002.

While it is possible for Ann to go to the corner shop, put a basket on her knee and get a few groceries, she cannot possibly do the weekly shop on her own: Dean has to accompany her. She is well aware that he'd much rather be kicking a football with his friends and feels badly that he has to spend Saturday morning going to the supermarket with his Mam, instead. It takes them about twenty minutes to get to the Square, Ann in her wheelchair and Dean walking by her side. 'I would never be able to do the weekly shop on my own because I wouldn't be able to manage a trolley or get stuff off the shelves. The barriers that are out there for people who are in wheelchairs are unbelievable – getting access to shops and other public buildings and getting access to a toilet, which is a basic need that everybody is entitled to. It's a total nightmare and so frustrating.'

In 2002 Ann became involved in DART Outreach – a voluntary group that lobbies TDs and county councillors, inviting them to accompany people in wheelchairs as they go about their business so that they can see how difficult it is to get around in a wheelchair. 'We are first class citizens, like anyone else, and we should be allowed to go anywhere we like – to the cinema, the shops, public toilets and so on. We're hopeful that things will improve, especially since 2003 is the Year of People with Disabilities.'

Despite the nightmarish barriers she meets everyday, Ann maintains a remarkably positive attitude to life. 'There's people an awful lot worse off than I am,' she says. 'I'm just another person, with a struggle in life, making the best of what I've got. And, in some ways, my life has totally changed for the better. I look younger now than I did when I was walking because I'm mixing with younger people. I wouldn't have said it a few years ago, but now I can say, "I love life." It's true.'

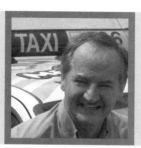

Pat Howe

... a taxi driver whose struggle to read and write led him to devise a board game that promotes literacy skills

PAT HOWE – A TAXI DRIVER FROM PALMERSTOWN, west Dublin – harbours an unusual ambition. Namely, to get into prison. He cannot wait for the day he can sit down with prisoners, particularly those who are illiterate, in order to play a board game he dreamed up several years ago.

Mentalogy was designed not just to be fun, but also to help those who struggle with reading and writing, as does a majority of the prison population. Pat himself knows what it is like to experience literacy problems: he received a rather haphazard education and it was not until he attended adult literacy classes at the age of twenty-seven that he really came to grips with reading and writing.

From the time of his 'very, very difficult' birth in 1950, the odds were stacked against Pat. The use of forceps during his long-drawn out delivery (he was in breech position) left him with clubfeet. And although, one year later, he could pull himself up into a standing position, it was impossible for him to put one foot in front of another because his feet were turned inwards to such an extent.

For the first two years of his life, his mum carried him in her arms everyday to Clontarf Orthopaedic Clinic to have dressings changed on his feet. At the age of three he had the first of many operations, during which the bones of his feet were broken and re-set. Each operation was followed by several months' recuperation in hospital. Pat's earliest memory is of learning to walk at two and a half with splints on his legs. He also remembers starting school when he was four, but two months later being brought to hospital for another operation. When he returned to the classroom six months later, he had fallen behind the rest of the class; further operations left him even further behind. 'I struggled to keep up,' he says. 'I'd kind of catch up and then I'd be back into hospital again. It was so frustrating.'

By the age of six he was wearing knee high boots that enabled him to join in games of football, as best he could. 'Most of the time my foot kicked the ground instead of the ball,' he says. 'A pair of shoes would last me about seven days and my mother was broke from buying me shoes. She bought me the best, but they still broke after a week because I made sure to do all the things kids want to do, like climbing trees.'

One day, when he was playing on the path outside his Cabra home, he overbalanced and stepped back onto the road, just as a ten-ton lorry was passing. 'The lorry ran over my right foot,' he says. 'The driver panicked and he reversed back over it. A quick-thinking neighbour ran out with a shovel, which she slid under the foot and used as a splint. Her daughter, who was about to get married, brought out some brand new towels she'd received as a wedding present and wrapped them around my foot.'

An ambulance took him to Temple Street Children's Hospital where doctors considered amputation. After all they had been through, however, Pat's mother insisted that the doctors at least try to save her son's foot, which they did. At the age of six, Pat had to learn to walk all over again. 'I didn't want anybody to see me; I felt a right bloody fool,' he says.

However, during his time in hospital he met an older boy, who had a profound impact on Pat. 'This guy, Richard, had polio and all he could do was move his head from side to side a little. Seeing him changed my life because it made me see how lucky I was and it made me realise I should never feel sorry for myself. I've never forgotten him and no matter what I've faced in life since then, I've said, "I'll get over this". Thinking of him encourages me to get out and do what I can.'

Pat had his last operation when he was eleven years old, by which time he had missed so much school that he still could not read. He could write, but his spelling was not great. 'It was so frustrating not being able to read, but I covered it up by memorising everything,' he says. 'My mother took it a bit easy on me and she never knew. When it came to doing my Primary Cert at the end of national school I couldn't read the questions. I put my hand up and told the supervisor I'd forgotten my glasses, so he would read the questions to me. I had memorised my English and Irish essays word for word and I was able to get them down on paper because I didn't care about the spelling. I barely passed. When I did the entrance exam for Cabra Tech I got zero because, again, I couldn't read the questions. I left school after the Group Cert.'

While his experience of education was clearly frustrating, Pat never lost sight of something his older brother, Eddie, said on a number of occasions. 'He was always saying things about me like, "That's a cute kid — he is so smart". That stuck with me and I'll always be grateful to him for that. And I was clever; I always knew I was clever. I didn't get a complex because I couldn't read or write; if anything, it made me more determined and I figured out ways of hiding it. I could commit things to memory and I was very good at maths because I found it easy to remember my tables.'

Pat found that having a good memory had definite advantages and, from the age of fourteen until he was eighteen, he 'made a fortune' from gambling. 'I never lost because I was able to read the cards so well,' he says, 'And I was terrific at looking at people and figuring out if they were bluffing. Everybody thought I was going to become a professional gambler, but at the age of eighteen I started working as a fitter and I never gambled again.'

When he was twenty-two Pat gave up his job to train full-time at kick-boxing, an extraordinary choice of sport for somebody who had endured numerous operations on his feet. He became 'so good and so fast' that, within eighteen months, he was picked to go and train in Thailand. However, he had recently met his wife-to-be, Therese, and they had decided to save up for a house and get married. He returned to his previous work as a fitter and married three years later. Therese was one of the few people he was honest with, regarding his difficulties with reading and writing. She was very understanding and encouraged him to attend adult literacy classes, which he started six months after their wedding. 'It turned out my reading and writing was better than I thought it was, but confidence is everything,' he says, 'I started picking up the newspaper and reading it every day. Then I started writing every day and I found I enjoyed it. I kept at it and, by the end of the year, I was grand. The only thing I have a phobia about now is having somebody watch me when I'm writing.'

When their two children, Gary and Nicole, came along, it was Therese who helped them with their homework. Nicole was a 'slow learner', but Pat encouraged her by saying, 'Keep it small, keep it simple: just learn a little bit at a time and don't worry about the big picture. Keep doing a little bit and then, one day, you'll wake up and you'll have the whole picture.' Nicole followed her father's advice and made steady progress at primary school and then at second level. In the end, she achieved four hundred points in her Leaving Certificate and she is now in her third year of science studies at Dublin City University. Gary did not find school a struggle; he has recently qualified as an electrician, but is actively pursuing a career in music.

Pat continues to believe in what he calls his 'daisy chain' method of memorising and in February 1999 he dreamt of a board game based on this concept which encourages the development of literacy skills. 'In my dream I was in a test and there were a series of cards and each one was lifted to show what was on it and put down again. It surprised me, but I could remember what was on each of them. I woke up in amazement and went, "Wow!" and then I fell instantly back to sleep. I got up the next morning and started building the game. And I've never looked back.'

Pat quit his job as a maintenance manager so that he could devote his time to fleshing out his concept. He put his memory to good use by taking the Public Service Vehicle test, which he passed first time. He then started working as a taxi driver, confident that he would soon meet somebody who would help him market his game. Sure enough, one day in December 1999 a graphic designer by the name of Pat Kinsley thumbed a lift. Pat told him of his idea and the pair spent the next couple of years developing Mentalogy the board game. Adopted by Neworld, the game was launched in April 2003 by the then Lord Mayor of Dublin, Councillor Dermot Lacey. Since then the game has been flying off the shelves of toyshops around the country. 'It has far exceeded our expectations,' says Mentalogy marketing director, David Conn. 'We expected it to sell in the hundreds in the first month of it going on sale, whereas it actually sold in the thousands.'

In Mentalogy players have to memorise cards containing words, numbers and images in order to progress around the board. 'It's a form of collective learning,' explains Pat. 'You start off with two or three cards and then you gradually increase the number. You can start by using the images and then progress onto the numbers and words. It helps people to memorise things. It's just a game, but with this game I'm trying to educate the world. We all have potential we haven't even tapped into: man's mind is unlimited, but it needs time to develop and learn. That's what my game is really all about – it's designed to help us exercise and expand our minds. The more we use our minds the more we learn, and the more we learn the more we realise there is to learn.'

Pat believes that education is 'the key to everything' and he has been delighted to see the effectiveness of his game at firsthand. He frequently gives demonstrations and during one, in Smyth's toyshop, Tallaght, a ten-year-old boy approached Pat and told him he had a poor attention span and that he was dyslexic. 'Within a couple of minutes he memorised nine image cards and I told him his concentration was fine,' says Pat. 'I moved onto the number cards and then the words. He got six out of nine right the first time, and then nine. He told me he was a terrible speller and I taught him to spell Mississippi in front of the crowd of people. He got a round of applause when he got it right. Can you imagine how he felt? I then got him to spell Mississippi backwards. Everyone gave him a big cheer and he told me, "You've blown my mind!"'

Pat was invited to the adult learning centre at Cherry Orchard to teach a woman who had left school at an early age without being able to write even her name. A teacher in her family had tried to help her read and write, but to no avail. 'She knew the letters of the alphabet, but she couldn't spell even simple two letter words,' says Pat. 'I took out my cards and asked her to memorise the spellings of two words, 'in' and 'to'. As her confidence increased I added another two cards and we continued like this until we got up to nineteen two-letter words and she could remember every single one. I called in her teacher and he couldn't believe it. He then started teaching her using the same method and, within weeks, she was writing full sentences without any spelling mistakes.'

Bernadette* says that Pat's 'daisy chain' method of learning has changed her life. Whereas she used to have to rely on her husband reading her letters out loud to her, she can now read them herself. 'Nothing seemed to register with me in school,' she says. 'I couldn't even write my own name I was that bad. And I couldn't spell Ballyfermot, where I live. Mentalogy is a fantastic game – it has completely changed my life – and I think it will bring many people a long way, especially people who can't

*Bernadette is not her real name.

read and write. It's helped my self-confidence and I've gone back to work recently, so it's opened a door for me that I won't let shut again. I could never play Monopoly with my kids because I couldn't read the words on the board, but now I can play it with them. I've only played Mentalogy at the adult learning centre, but I'm hoping to get my own game for my fortieth birthday. I'd love to introduce it to the kids because I know they'd have great fun with it.'

It has been exciting for Pat to walk into shops and see his game on the shelves, but he gets an even greater thrill seeing the effect the game sometimes has on people. 'I love meeting people and I love seeing their self-confidence increasing,' he says. 'That's the real reward. I'm not doing this for fame. Sure, I love it when someone comes up to me and says, "Great game!" – I get a buzz out of that – but that's not what it's about. The real reward comes in seeing my friend's twelve-year-old child, who has learning difficulties, learn to read and write and to speak properly within months of learning by my method. He's gone from being a quiet child to being confident and outgoing.'

Other countries, including the USA, have expressed interest in marketing Mentalogy and people are telling Pat that he is set to become a rich man. But he is no more interested in money than he is in fame and he fully intends to set up a trust fund for the homeless, alcoholics and drug addicts. Half of the proceeds from his game will be channelled into this fund. 'I understand that money is power, so I want to use the money for good,' says Pat. 'I am already comfortable – I have a nice house and car – and I don't need anything more than that.

'The more successful Mentalogy becomes, the more humble I have to become. I'm blessed by what's happened to me and I wouldn't change one second of my life because everything that's happened – all the pain and all the misery of my early years – has made me who I am. I wouldn't be who I am if I hadn't had all those experiences – all the ups and all the downs. My life has been exciting – even learning to walk was exciting. Twice! I know now why I went through what I did and I realise why I was born onto this planet – it was to give this game as a gift to the world and to make it successful. I believe that everything that's happened in my life has led up to it.

'What can you take with you when you die? You can only take one thing and that is happiness: you can either die happy or you can die miserable. I intend to die happy and helping people is what makes me happy. At the end of the day, money means nothing. Sure, I need money to live and the more money I have the quicker I can get around to change the world.'

Pat speaks like a man with a mission. 'I know where I'm going and I know what I'm doing,' he asserts. 'I need to build an awareness of what I'm trying to achieve through the game and I'm delighted that I've been invited to speak to business studies students at Trinity and DCU and psychology students at Ohio State University. I'm also looking forward to talking to primary school teachers about the game; I think that will be my proudest moment.

'I hope my story will inspire people to follow their dreams and that the board game will help countless people realise theirs. I'm trying to say to people, "Whatever gifts you're given, maximise them", and when I look back on my life I think I've maximised my gifts beyond my wildest dreams. And I'm not saying that in a boastful way. I'm not trying to be a saint because I'm not a saint; I am simply trying not to be a sinner. When I die I would like to see on my tombstone, "Here lies a good man – he did his best." And I know everybody in the world can aspire to that.'

Anyone who hails a bright yellow Dublin taxi with the word Mentalogy emblazoned across it should be prepared! Not only will they be treated to an entertaining and informative conversation, ranging from philosophy and religion to Pat's vision of a car-free capital city, they will also have the opportunity to buy their very own signed edition of the driver's unique board game. Never one to miss an opportunity, Pat always keeps a couple of his games in the car.

'I know what my future is,' says Pat. 'I know what I have to do — continue to reach people, to give them hope. I am excited at the thought of how many people the game is going to reach. Of course I am! Eighty per cent of the prison population can't read and write and I'd love to get into prison. That's my ambition. I've tried, but I've met nothing but closed doors up until now. I haven't given up, though. I know it will happen some day — when the time is right.'

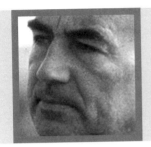

Samuel Malcolmson

... who has had an IRA bullet lodged in his spine
for thirty years and who founded the Disabled
Police Officers' Association

SAMUEL MALCOLMSON FROM KATESBRIDGE, Co. Down, had everything to live for in the early 1970s. A young police officer with the Royal Ulster Constabulary, he and his girlfriend, Gayus, were planning to move to Canada where he would join the Mounties and Gayus would find work as a physiotherapist. That was the plan.

However, love's young dream was shattered one night in September 1972 when Officer Malcolmson was going about his duties on a dark, lonely road in south Armagh. He had gone with a colleague to investigate the shooting of a soldier when the car, in which he was a front seat passenger, came under attack from two IRA gunmen. One bullet smashed through a window and lodged itself in the young officer's lower spine. Another struck the driver in the back. 'He slumped forward over the steering wheel while the car was still moving,' remembers Samuel. 'And a memory that still haunts me is the fear that we wouldn't be able to drive any further and the gunmen would simply walk up to the car and shoot us like dogs.'

Somehow, with Samuel helping to steer, the two RUC men managed to return to base — and to safety. 'We were weaving across the road the three or four miles back to base,' says Samuel, 'And when we got there, we smashed into a wall. I was screaming my head off with pain — the army gave us morphine while we waited for the ambulance to come from Newry. It was like a nightmare.'

Samuel soon slipped into unconsciousness and the fact that he was given the last rites shows just how close he came to 'packing it all in'. He was airlifted the next day to the Royal Victoria Hospital, Belfast where he spent the next nine months. Only close family was allowed to visit, but Gayus managed to slip in unnoticed each evening (the physiotherapist's uniform she wore for work at the City Hospital successfully fooled staff into thinking she was working at the Royal).

For months Samuel could not understand why his mother did not visit him until, finally, his minister took him by the hand one day and broke the shocking news to him — his dear mother had died of shock at his bedside the day after the shooting. The fact that his family had to suffer is something Samuel has never come to terms with. 'As a policeman I accepted I might be injured, but one thing I'll never forgive the IRA men for is that someone else in my family had to die,' he says. 'I wonder did the gunman who shot me think that getting my mother was a bonus? I wonder did he even think twice about what he did?'

The bullet, which shattered into pieces and lodged in his lower spine, left Samuel with his left leg paralysed and chronic pain in his right leg. Just walking from his house to the car is sheer agony for him. It was an experience that could have left the young man consumed with bitterness and self-pity, as he struggled to come to terms with his disability. But Samuel Malcolmson is not that kind of person. He determined to make the most of his circumstances, telling himself that 'disability is not inability'.

Ten years after his accident he became a founding member of the Disabled Police Officers' Association (DPOA). The majority of members, like Samuel, had been discharged from the RUC on medical grounds as a consequence of injuries sustained as the result of terrorism. In its early days the association sold numerous badges to raise funds and promote awareness and in 1987 Samuel became chairman, a position he held for the next ten years. As chairman, his primary concern was to encourage the 160 members to lead as normal lives as possible, including getting out and about and enjoying a range of sports and hobbies. 'Some people came out of hospital and sat in a corner doing nothing, being a nuisance to their wives,' he says. 'I thought there was no point in heaping sympathy on them and I tried to get them back into the mainstream of life. I told them that disability throws down a challenge – it does not mean inability.'

Counselling was an important aspect of his role as chairman. 'The phone never stopped ringing,' he says. 'People would ring at all times of day and night because they just wanted someone to talk to. It helps if you've been there yourself – because I'm disabled myself, I can tell someone to get off their backside and take up a sport or hobby. A huge number of people said that the committee of the DPOA were better counsellors than anyone else because we really listened to people and we had been through similar circumstances. I got the feeling that some disabled policemen were sitting on a time bomb, by keeping in their grief, and that some day the whole thing was going to explode. Two members committed suicide.'

Once a keen sportsman – his hobbies had included cross-country running and stock car racing – Samuel knew what struggling to come to terms with a lack of mobility was like. Following his accident he took up discus and javelin and, along with six other members, took part in the Games for the Disabled in Swindon in 1994. 'We just jumped in with both feet – in some cases, no feet – and decided to give it a go,' he says. For one man, a paraplegic who for twenty years had sat slumped in his wheelchair, it proved a transforming experience. 'It was like a miracle, watching him,' says Samuel. 'It was amazing the way it showed it's a case of mind over matter.'

During the event DPOA members were shocked to discover that limb replacements in Great Britain were far more sophisticated than those on offer in Northern Ireland. 'Athletes on the mainland were years ahead in the quality of their limbs,' says Samuel. 'We were competing against men with state of the art limbs while our members were using limbs that could be seen in World War One films.'

Although he never needed an artificial limb himself, Samuel undertook to campaign for better quality limbs to be made available in Northern Ireland. This was one of a number of issues the DPOA acted on as a pressure group. They reckoned that good quality limbs were not being approved for use in Northern Ireland because of the expense. One member forked out £8,000 to buy a set of sophisticated limbs in the US, only to discover there was nowhere in Northern Ireland he could have them serviced. 'We've always been a group looking for the best for its members,' says Samuel. 'Everything we needed became a fight: every time we wanted to get noticed we had to put some kind of controversial report in the newspapers. Nothing was simply handed to us.'

The DPOA also campaigned for better treatment of policemen who had been injured in the line of duty. This resulted in a policy of greater numbers of maimed officers being kept on in the RUC to carry out light duties; it also resulted in better compensation than before. Samuel had received compensation of £40,000. 'At that time that was a good reward,' he says. 'But, looking back now, I wish I had never accepted a medical discharge. I was living in Newcastle then and I was told that the only work for me would have been in one of the headquarter stations in Belfast, which would have been an hour and a half's drive to and from work. I didn't receive any advice and I thought £40,000 was good. We bought our house outright and we watched the money gradually go down, down, down, until ten years later it was all gone. My colleague, who was driving the car when we came under fire, lost a lung, but recovered enough to continue in the RUC; he went on to become an inspector.'

That was over thirty years ago now. 'I can honestly say that in all that time I have been in constant pain,' says Samuel. 'It starts in my lower back and goes down over the hip and right down the outside of my left leg and into the toes. It is like severe sciatic pain and it just keeps running up and down my leg. Sometimes the only way I can cope is to get offside — to lock myself in the bedroom. I have four daughters — Joanne, Andrea, Gail and Nicola — and it hasn't been fair on them that I spend so much time in the bedroom, but it is the only way I can cope. I can't mix with them and control the pain at the same time because I am like a bear with a sore head.

'When they were younger and we went to the beach or to Tollymore Forest Park, I would sit in the car reading newspapers because I couldn't walk even fifty yards without being in pain. That was very hard because a lot of bringing up kids involves chasing them around, climbing trees and running in and out of the sea with them. It really hurt watching other dads play with their kids; I felt jealous of them. Quite a few of the DPOA members said they found that one of the hardest things — not being able to get involved in the rough and tumble of daily family life.

'Gayus has always said that I have built a wall around myself that nobody can get over. And I would agree. I think you do it because you don't want your family suffering what you're suffering, so you choose to suffer behind a wall. But then your family feels excluded. The number of times Gayus used to ask me, "Can I help you?" and I'd say abruptly, "No, just leave me." The kids learned when to leave me alone. It hurts me to say that, but it's true.'

Chronic pain turned Samuel into a different kind of person and he didn't expect Gayus to stick with him. At the time of his accident, her parents were moving from Zambia to New Zealand and he urged her to join them. But she had no intention of leaving him, even though their plans of moving to Canada had been hopelessly dashed. They married in

1974. 'Even though we weren't engaged at the time of his accident, we were very close and I had no intention of leaving him,' says Gayus. 'But he did have a personality change as a result of his injury. He used to be such an outgoing, happy-go-lucky character, but there's some days now I wouldn't go near him.

'As the years go on, he's become more reclusive than ever. He's really not comfortable anywhere other than home and, even at home, he spends an awful lot of time on his own. I could honestly say that the number of evenings he comes and sits in the living room are very few and far between. And, if he does, he doesn't stay for more than an hour. We seldom go out because he doesn't like being in crowded places. He'll drive me to the shops, but he won't come in; he waits in the car because he just can't cope. We've lost touch with a lot of people and it's left us very isolated. I would have liked to return to work part-time after we'd had the children, but I couldn't have left Samuel at home to look after the girls. The way he tenses up with pain, he couldn't have managed. I've always understood why he has to retreat to the bedroom; I know he just has to be away on his own.'

Another aspect of the DPOA's work that Samuel undertook was campaigning for the improvement of Northern Ireland's pain clinics. 'There's always been pain clinics, but they have never received enough funding,' he says. 'There was a time, if you were overcome by pain, you could have knocked on the door of a pain clinic and got a nerve block injection almost immediately, but that ended. It became a case of ringing up and seeing when they could fit you in. You might have had to wait a month, which was so crazy when you were in chronic pain. Over the years I met many government officials, civil servants and Secretaries of State and even Prince Charles, but the only person who made any real difference was Michael Mates, the Conservative MP. It was he who brought it back to the situation whereby you could get treatment immediately if you needed it. Sir Kenneth Bloomfield made a difference, too. When he wrote up his report for the Millennium Fund there was a brief mention made of chronic pain sufferers and I thought there would only be a small amount of money. But in fact it worked out well. Anybody who suffers chronic pain can receive £1,000 to see a consultant and get an assessment of their pain; they can apply for further money, if it is needed.'

As a result of the Millennium Fund, Samuel and others who suffer chronic pain can apply for the £7,000 it costs to receive a spinal implant. It works on the same principle as a TENS machine: it is a non-destructive means of interrupting pain signals (by substituting small electrical signals for pain signals going to the brain). Samuel was on a waiting list to undergo a spinal implant operation at the Causeway Hospital, Coleraine, until the doctor realised this would not be possible due to an infection around the bullet. Dr Cooper suggested, instead, that he could place the machine in Samuel's upper hip – a procedure that has never been tried before. 'I am happy to be a guinea pig,' says Samuel. 'It will not be as difficult a procedure as a spinal implant because it will not be as critical: he can't paralyse my leg because it's already paralysed. And, who knows, maybe it will be a first and it will work!

'Some of my vertebrae were badly shattered by the bullet and three of them fused together. The doctors never figured out why my spinal cord wasn't actually severed – the bullet disintegrated and bits and pieces flew off in different directions. The reason I had to lie on my back in hospital for so many months was to allow the bones to fuse together. The implant will not be a cure as such, but it will allow me to help control the pain; I'll be able to control it by switching on the machine and controlling the frequency. I've a friend who had a spinal implant operation and he says it gives him relief for a couple of hours after he uses it, which is good.'

Samuel currently takes at least twenty-four tablets a day in an attempt to control his pain. 'I take six tablets four times a day – morphine, Neuronton and Solpadeine – and, recently, I've been waking at night and taking an extra dose. At times, I also take anti-inflammatory tablets for my lower back. I feel the pain is getting worse and I often ask my doctor, "Is there nothing new I can try?" If there's something new on the market

I always want to try it; I don't mind being a guinea pig. And I don't mind admitting that I sometimes experiment with other people's drugs.

'Cannabis is supposed to be good for pain and I did get some grass at one stage to give it a go. We've four children in the house and we're always saying to them not to get involved with drugs and so I went down to the end of the yard to smoke my first joint. After I took a few drags I felt a tingling sensation in every nerve ending and the pain was gone, but when I tried to walk back to the house I couldn't put one foot in front of the other. Well, my left leg doesn't work anyway, but I couldn't get my right leg to move forward. I don't know what happened, but I ended up coming back to the house hand over hand – crawling! Can you imagine if any of the girls had seen me? After that I smoked in the bedroom, but after a while it was hard to get grass – I could only get cannabis resin. I remember getting a severe throat infection one time – the resin must have been laced with something else – and I never touched it again. It was only recently my eldest daughter, Joanne, said to me something about the sweet smells that used to come from the bedroom. I used to pass it off as pot pourri, but it turns out she knew rightly!'

Samuel walks with a stick and his lack of stability means that he is prone to falls. Twice, when he has fallen, he has broken his kneecap; another time he broke the femur in his left leg.

His chronic pain is a constant and cruel reminder of the day an IRA gunman shattered not just Samuel's lower vertebrae, but also his dream of a future in the Canadian Mounties. It is not something he can easily forget. 'There were two gunmen and they were never caught,' he says, 'But I'm convinced I know who they are. Two people were brought in, but they were released without charge because there was no proof. One person who lived in the area was able to identify them, but he didn't want to make himself a target by coming forward.

'Have you ever had a question that's gnawed away at you?' he continues. 'Something you would love to find out? The gunman knows who he is –

I was his enemy and he shot me. I would simply love to ask him, "When you heard that my mother dropped dead at my bedside the day after you shot me, did you feel any sense of remorse? Were you truly sorry that happened? Or were you sitting in a pub somewhere saying to yourself that was good because you'd got two for the price of one?" That question is never out of my mind and I often think of seeking out the individual and asking him that.

'There's been lots of occasions when gunmen have shot themselves or blown themselves up. To me, that is justice — if they lived by the sword, it's only just that they die by the sword. But I know that these guys who fired shots at me are still around and I'd just love to know, when the news broke that my mother had died at my bedside, how they reacted. I will never rest easy until I know the answer to that question.'

So long as Samuel Malcolmson continues to suffer chronic pain from the bullet lodged in his lower spine, how can he and his wife, Gayus, possibly be expected to forget the night the Irish Republican Army shattered love's young dream?

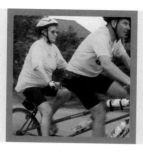

Rita Corley

*... who became a plucky adventurer and fundraiser
after she was blinded in a car crash*

RITA CORLEY CAN JUST ABOUT REMEMBER what her four children look like. It is fourteen years since she last saw them, even though they all live within easy reach of her home in Milltown, south Dublin. Her youngest son, Vincent, was just five years old the last time she set eyes on him; she can only imagine what he looks like now that he's a young man.

Rita has not seen any of her five grandchildren either. It is not that she is disinterested in her family. Far from it! Like any mother or grandmother, she loves being involved in the lives of her children and grandchildren – chatting with them and hearing about their latest interests. And, like any proud mum, she accompanied her daughters, Lisa and Geraldine, when they went shopping for their wedding dresses (they both got married in 1995). However, a day that is filled with joy for most mothers proved traumatic for Rita. 'Trying to act like a normal mum was very tough,' she recalls.

It had never crossed her mind when the girls were growing up that she would be denied the pleasure of seeing them in all their bridal glory. She had always loved clothes and colour and shopping, but these simple pleasures were cruelly wrenched from her grasp in the early hours of 12 October 1989. Driving home from The Goat Grill, where she worked as a waitress, Rita was involved in a head-on collision. In a single moment, that was to change her life forever, the lights were switched off for Rita. She has inhabited a place of darkness ever since – a world in which a bright summer's day is as black as the darkest, moonless night. Rita's busy life as a mother, a waitress and a voluntary worker was turned upside down in an instant.

She had been cruising along in her car, 'as happy as can be', as she thought about the great buzz there had been in the pub that night. Ireland had qualified for the European Cup by beating Northern Ireland and, before starting work, she had purchased a ticket to fly out to Australia to be with daughter Lisa on her twenty-first birthday. There was little traffic on the roads at that hour and Rita only vaguely remembers a milk float coming towards her on the wrong side of the road. She expected it to pull up onto the path, but it didn't.

'Next thing there was a bang,' she recalls. 'I got out to see if anybody was hurt, but I just collapsed on the road. With the impact of the crash, the glass of the windscreen had come in on top of me and gone right into my eyes. When I got to hospital the surgeon said she might be able to save fifty per cent of the sight in one of my eyes and, when I woke up in the after care ward, I asked a young nurse how the operation went. She said, "Great! Everything went wonderful", so I thought I still had one eye left. But I had none. It turned out both eyes had to be removed because they were cut behind and there would have been no hope of a transplant.'

The next day Rita's husband, Eamonn, rang Lisa, who immediately flew home from Australia. 'He didn't tell Lisa the extent of the damage,' says Rita, 'But over a cup of coffee at the airport Vincent told her, "Mam will never see again". She lost her head and the whole family went to pieces: everybody was very upset and my mother, who was living with us at the time, went wild.'

Rita was in hospital for three months, during which time she put on a brave face. A social worker from the National Council for the Blind of Ireland (NCBI) visited her and, once Rita was discharged, came to see her at home. She suggested Rita get a guide dog – a suggestion Rita immediately dismissed because her mother had once been bitten by a dog. However, she found she did not like using a cane. 'I got training in how to use it and the teachers were excellent,' she says, 'But every time I went out and banged a cane, I felt I lost my dignity.'

In the end, she had a 'good chat' with her Mam, who saw the sense in Rita getting a guide dog. So Rita went on the waiting list with the Irish Guide Dogs For The Blind; it was a couple of years later that she got her first dog, Breffni. In the meantime, Rita was well looked after at home. Her mother, Esther Quinn, would not even let her fill a kettle. 'I was very spoiled,' Rita remembers. 'My daughters were still living at home – Lisa was twenty-one and Geraldine was nineteen – and they did everything for me. In hindsight now, I think I would have preferred to have gone straight into a course and become more independent from the beginning.'

Before she was allowed to take Breffni home, Rita had to spend a month receiving training at the association's headquarters in Cork. Even though she 'cried solidly' the first week, her misery paid off when she finally arrived back in Dublin. 'I came home on my own on the train with the dog and, when I was met at the train station, there was great excitement. Breffni was a beauty – half labrador and half retriever – and he had a lovely temperament. He made an enormous difference to my life. I missed him dreadfully when he had to retire, but now I have a golden labrador, Larch, and I go to the shops, the hairdressers, the bank and to church with him.'

Having a dog is 'fantastic', but unfortunately does not guarantee a safe journey, especially when the paths are 'in such a dreadful way'. One day when Rita was crossing the road, Breffni suddenly stopped. Thinking they had reached the kerb, Rita said, 'Up'. 'I didn't know there was a hole in the road – Breffni went down and I went down. I was in bits – my face was badly scarred – and I lost my confidence. I didn't go out again for months.'

Rita has tried her best to adapt to being blind, but she frequently experiences frustrations in her daily life. For example, whenever she tries to do the dusting, she finds herself knocking over ornaments. These days it is Eamonn who does much of the work around the house. A bus driver, he does not start work until the afternoon. While he's at work, Rita does what she can to prepare dinner – usually peeling the vegetables, which she asks Eamonn to check when he arrives home. 'I'm still quite scared of cooking,' she says. 'I'd be scared of pots boiling over and things like that, but I don't mind peeling the vegetables, once someone checks them. I have everything organised and ready for Eamonn to cook when he comes in at eight-thirty. It means we eat quite late and one thing I'm looking forward to, when Eamonn retires, is eating earlier.

'As the years go on I don't find it getting any easier. Although I've accepted my blindness now, I still have very bad days. You can kind of adapt yourself, but it can be very frustrating when you keep banging into things in your own home and you can never look out the window at the garden and watch it changing with the different seasons. When you're totally in the dark, it's black, black all the time. I miss a lot of things, especially seeing the faces of my children, and I'd love to be able to see my grandchildren. I used to love shopping, but I don't bother now – the girls do most of it for me – although sometimes they'll insist on bringing me with them, say, to Liffey Valley. They'll say to me, "Mam, instead of lying on the bed, you're coming with us!" and they'll try to involve me.'

Rita misses her work at The Goat Grill 'dreadfully'. Until her accident, she had worked there for nearly seven years and, before that, she spent eleven years working in the Burlington Hotel. Although she no longer works there, the owner of The Goat Grill, Charlie Chawke, has been 'very good' to her and she often goes there on fundraising missions, usually selling raffle tickets. In fact, Rita has become something of an expert when it comes to fundraising.

Her children call her 'a professional beggar' — a description to which she does not object.

'It's something I have to do,' she says. 'In the early days I thought I'd end up in a mental home or I'd become an alcoholic and I think getting involved in fundraising helped me avoid going down either of those roads. I want to raise funds for the NCBI and the Irish Guide Dogs For the Blind because they both helped me after I had my accident.

'I've made a lot of friends through the NCBI and I meet up with them every Tuesday at the headquarters, Iona House. Some have been blind since birth and they are very independent — they put me to shame, really. They've never known any other way and they got proper training, as children, at St Mary's or St Joseph's. Others lost their sight at an early age and sometimes I think to myself, "At least I had my sight for forty-six years".

'It's very hard to change your lifestyle, though. I really miss driving. Even though my husband's a bus driver, I was never on a bus really; I drove everywhere. And I never had any time for walking because I was working as well as looking after my family and my mother. I had a very busy life. Sometimes I get a bus now, but not very much because getting on a bus with a guide dog is an ordeal. I tried to learn Braille in the beginning, but I couldn't adapt to it. Now, if I'm having a bad evening, I just go up to bed and listen to the radio or to a tape. I used to read the likes of Catherine Cookson and Danielle Steele and I can get their books on tape.'

Rita admits she sometimes feels sorry for herself and asks, 'Why me?' She says, 'At times I've been angry with God; sometimes I've asked myself is there a God at all. I used to help others by delivering meals on wheels and bringing old people to hospital and I can't do any of that now. But then I think of the wonderful people I have met through the NCBI and the Irish Guide Dogs For The Blind.'

Not only has the loss of her sight meant that her circle of friends has greatly widened, but it has also opened up a whole new world of challenges and adventures. Rita has undertaken an extraordinary range of fundraising trips with the NCBI, including canoeing and tandem-riding in the US, skiing in Austria and tandem-riding and mountain climbing in Thailand. 'Thailand was a wonderful experience, but it was tough; at one stage we had to go over a river on a rope and we'd had no practice beforehand. Our leader, Eamonn Duffy, used to say each morning, "Now, this is going to be a very easy day" and, at the beginning, I was very innocent and I believed him. But it would end up being the toughest day ever and I'd be going mad! Even during the cycling trip he'd say, "Now there's no hills today" and we'd get to the biggest hill we could ever meet: we'd have to get off the bikes and walk, the hill was that steep.'

During a canoeing trip in 'alligator territory' in north Florida, Rita had to face head-on her deep-rooted fear of water. Not to mention her fear of alligators! As it happened, the only alligator spotted by any member of the group was a dead one lying on the riverbank. 'The stench from it was something awful! We ate alligator meat one night, which I enjoyed until I discovered what it was. One day one of my friends, who is also blind, toppled over in her canoe and ended up in the water. I think I would have gone hysterical if that had happened to me. I'm terrified of water — before I lost my sight I went for private swimming lessons in an attempt to get over my fear, but I just could not take to it. I hate water hitting my face — I even prefer a bath to a shower because of it.'

These fund-raising trips are by no means holidays. For a start, they usually involve getting up at four-thirty or five o'clock in the morning. On each trip a sighted friend has accompanied Rita, but no one has ever wanted to go a second time because 'it's all hard work'. Since the trips are all about fundraising, Rita does not mind this: she likes to cover as much ground (or water) as possible — whether by bicycle, ski, canoe or on foot. 'I think when you're doing a challenge — when you're really doing it for a cause — you like to do as many miles as possible. We'd be up early before the hot sun and then we'd go out again in the afternoon.'

In 2002 Rita did not go abroad, but chose instead to do a parachute jump in Edenderry, Co. Offaly. 'It was nerve-racking, but my tandem-pilot, a young lad called Roger, was absolutely wonderful. He guided me down. I tried to remember everything I had been told, like keeping my two feet up, and I landed with a bump on my bottom. My husband said it was absolutely amazing to see me drifting down. There were a few other people tandem jumping that day, one of whom broke their ankle; I was the only person who was blind.'

The parachute jump did not bring in as much money as any of her trips, but Rita has now raised an incredible total of £36,000 for the NCBI. She has lost track of how much she has raised for the Irish Guide Dogs For The Blind through church collections, hampers, calendars and Christmas cards. She finds fundraising is becoming increasingly difficult with more and more charities 'out there' competing with each other. She often involves local children in door-to-door collections and raffles and, from time to time, shows her appreciation by throwing a party for them.

As for her own financial situation, Rita is happy enough to get by on her blind pension. She did receive a certain amount of compensation from the company that owned the milk float her car collided with, but she gave this to members of her family. 'I'm quite happy to sit back now and just have my blind pension, but to get it I had to go before a panel of social welfare officers, so they could assess if I was really blind (my husband went mad about that).

'At the end of the day no amount of money could make up for the loss of my sight. Not at all. I'd have been happy to have had one eye left and have got no money; I would love just to be able to tell night from day. I don't blame the driver of the milk float, though. It was just a freak accident and I wouldn't mind meeting him to tell him I've no hard feelings against him.'

Rita turns sixty soon and she would like to celebrate her birthday with some kind of unusual fundraising venture, although she has yet to decide what that might be. 'I've thought and thought a lot about it; I'd love to do something special.'

As for the future, one thing is certain: Rita will be taking part in many more fundraising challenges. 'It's the challenges and the fundraising trips that have helped keep me going,' she says. 'I really do enjoy them. And that's why I keep going back for more.'

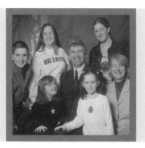

The Ryan Family

... who find that having a child with a disability has greatly enriched their lives

MICHAEL AND TERESA RYAN of Pallasgrean, Co. Limerick received their best Christmas present ever in 1991. After spending almost two months in Our Lady's Hospital for Sick Children, Dublin, they were finally allowed to return home on Christmas Eve with their thirteen-month-old daughter, Ríona, who, only weeks earlier, had come through major heart surgery by the skin of her teeth.

Three days after the operation they had been woken up in the middle of the night by a nurse, saying, 'I'm sorry, I'm sorry.' Ríona's heart had stopped beating and Michael and Teresa had to wait in a nearby room while medical staff frantically worked on reviving her. So it was with great joy that the Ryans finally returned home with their bundle of joy, and were reunited with the rest of the family for the festive celebrations. Her two sisters, Anna-Jane and Úna, were waiting anxiously to welcome her home, as was her brother, Eamon.

It had been a traumatic thirteen months for Michael and Teresa, who met in the early 1980s when they were both working as volunteers at a social club for people with learning disabilities. As a result of their years of involvement with people with disabilities, it was only natural that they would ask the question 'What if?' during Teresa's first couple of pregnancies. By the time she was pregnant with Ríona, however, they had stopped asking the question. As it happened, Ríona was born with Down Syndrome and profound deafness.

Her heart defect was discovered the day after her birth and it was this that most preoccupied her parents. Even after her operation there were a number of times when Ríona was at death's door. 'It took a good few years for her to get over the surgery,' says Teresa. 'She got pneumonia and collapsed a few times and there were a lot of times when she nearly died on us, so her first few years were very traumatic for us. She also had damaged lungs and it took a while for them to regenerate. We had a number of scares and we had to bring her to hospital quite a few times.'

Michael and Teresa reacted differently to the knowledge that their fourth child had a disability – two disabilities, in fact. Teresa, who by that time had spent thirteen years working as a nurse with adults with learning disabilities, immediately wondered what the future would hold for Ríona. 'I kept thinking of the lack of services for adults with intellectual disabilities,' she says. 'I was looking far down the road from day one because I'd seen all the hurt, the rejection and the lack of acceptance that people are sometimes subjected to by the public. On the other hand, because our lives had revolved around people with intellectual disabilities, we had a deep sense of commitment and affection for them, which meant the foundation was already there. There was no sense of rejection from either of us; we couldn't reject our own flesh and blood. For me, however, there was a sadness – it wasn't that I was rejecting Ríona, I loved her to pieces – but there was a sadness that used to fill up inside me when I tried to imagine what her future would be like. Over time I stopped looking twenty years down the road and I learned to take each day as it came. I realised we couldn't plan; we could only hope for the best.'

Michael, on the other hand, was immediately struck by the irony of the situation. 'It was really quite ironic, given that Teresa and I had met through disability,' he says. 'But this was very different because, up until then, disability had always been at a distance – it hadn't impinged on our family life. It was a different thing altogether to have someone with a disability in our own home. It was a little bit traumatic because we were expecting a healthy baby, but I never felt that it was something I needed to come to terms with. I remember someone rang and said, "I'm sorry for your troubles" and I found that strange because I didn't feel that Ríona was, in any sense, trouble.'

Teresa, meanwhile, wondered why she was receiving no cards or flowers, as she had following the births of her other children. It was only when word got out as to how positive Michael and Teresa were feeling about the birth of Ríona – they did not see it as a major tragedy – that the cards and gifts began to arrive. When they brought her home from hospital they did not tell her siblings that there was anything different about her. It was only when they came into the house one day, after playing outside, that they asked, 'Is Ríona handicapped?' One of their playmates had obviously said that to them, but Teresa's response was to sit them down and tell them that they were not to use that word. 'I told them that I didn't like the word "handicapped" and that I didn't want to hear them using it,' she says. 'I then explained to them that Ríona would need a lot of help and attention and that she would be a lot slower than themselves.'

The Ryans determined not to differentiate too much between Ríona and her siblings, apart from when it came to her medical needs. Inevitably, she needed a great deal of attention during her first few years: she was often sickly and her developmental progress was greatly delayed. In fact, she reached many of her milestones at roughly the same time as her younger sister, Maria, who arrived when Ríona was three. Despite intensive physiotherapy sessions, she made no effort to walk until Maria did. Only then did she give up on bum-shuffling, which she had found a perfectly satisfactory means of getting around (one time, when she was four, she escaped from her home and made her way, on her bottom, to the local shop). This was a very stressful period for the Ryans. 'Essentially, we had two babies,' says Teresa. 'We had to bring two buggies everywhere we went and then we had three older children to keep an eye on as well. That was a difficult time. The support of family and friends became very important, as did the devoted care and love of our childminder, Joan Clifford.'

Ríona, who is now thirteen, has progressed in leaps and bounds. She has a cheery, outgoing personality and is well able to hold her own at home and at school (she has attended the Midwest School for Deaf Children since she was seven). 'She's well able to assert herself inside and outside the family and well able to make friends,' says Teresa. 'When we go out, she always tries to break away from the family and make her own friends. Sometimes we worry that other kids might make fun of her, but that hasn't happened. Other children are usually fascinated by her use of sign language and they try to figure out what she's saying to them. She has a terrific memory and, if you bring her somewhere, she'll always remember the way. She's given us a couple of frights: once or twice, while on camping holidays in France, she has gone off on her own to the playground or the swimming pool. While this would not be unusual for a child of her age, we have to constantly watch her because she has no sense of danger.'

Ríona is 'a regular youngster' who loves television, dolls, cards and shopping. 'She is very vulnerable, but she is also a very sensitive and gifted child,' says Teresa. 'If one of us is feeling down or upset, she immediately senses it and gives us affection. She senses the need. If somebody hurts themselves, she immediately goes over and tries to help them out.'

Michael says they have always tried to treat Ríona in the same manner as her siblings. 'They are very good with her,' he says. 'They're mad about her and she's mad about them. They just treat her normally — they fight with her and they love her, just like any brothers and sisters. We have found it a great blessing to have somebody with a disability in our family, just as we've discovered the great blessing it has been to have each of our other children in the family. Ríona is so open towards everyone she meets and people are always drawn towards her. There's no doubt about that. I think people in Ireland, particularly older people, are very drawn towards people with disabilities. Ríona has a lovely smile and, when we're walking along in shopping centres, people will always smile at her. Some children with disabilities are very difficult to manage, but we've been lucky with Ríona – she's really quite placid – and she often sits quietly with a book or with her playing cards. We're fortunate in that regard because some children with learning disabilities just don't stay still – they're on the move all the time – and that's very difficult for the parents because it's never-ending. It can be very tough for them.'

Although the Ryans have not found having a child with a disability particularly difficult, their hearts go out to those who do find it a struggle. 'In recent years I have become mindful of the fact that there can be a lot of pain around having a child with a disability – a lot of pain – particularly if the child is the firstborn,' says Michael. 'I do sense a lot of suffering sometimes when I meet other parents of children with disabilities. It's important for other people to be aware of that and to acknowledge that it can be very difficult for parents. We know that a lot of parents do feel it and feel it terribly; they find it very, very difficult to accept. We are aware of that and we do acknowledge that it's not all sweetness and light. We did have difficult days early on and it does change family life – it changes everything, really.'

Michael, who trained as a primary school teacher and has a Masters in Religious Education, was principal of St Kieran's, Limerick, for ten years. Now an RE adviser for the primary schools of the diocese of Limerick, his role is to encourage and support the faith formation of the children of the diocese. He visits schools throughout the diocese, including a number for children with physical and learning disabilities. He is also a member of a special education sub-committee of the National

Association of Primary Diocesan Advisers, which was formed partly in response to the designation of 2003 as the European Year of People with Disabilities as well as the hosting of the Special Olympics World Summer Games in Ireland for the first time. The Ryans also played a part in this latter event by hosting two 'super' athletes from Kyrgyzstan in their home, an experience that they found highly enriching. They were glad that the event brought recognition to the abilities of people with intellectual difficulties. 'It was a huge and very successful community effort in Pallasgrean and it highlighted the needs of people with disabilities,' says Michael. 'And that can only be good.'

Teresa's work with the Brothers of Charity Services, Bawnmore, involves bringing the attention of the wider community to the needs of people with learning disabilities. 'In my work I've always been very aware of promoting the rights of people with disabilities – seeing their abilities first, not their disabilities,' she says. 'A lot of my work is about advocacy and, after Ríona was born, I became even more of an advocate for people with disabilities; I became more conscious of the person and their abilities rather than of the disability. Every year, for example, we have a service-user conference, which is run by people with intellectual disabilities. I find that parents of adults with disabilities may sometimes relate well to me when they know that I have a child with a disability too, because I've no fears about sharing my own experiences with them.

'Obviously there's still a lot to be done in Irish society to ensure that people with disabilities are seen as people first. It's only in the last three or four years that things have started to move in that direction. Ireland is now moving away from institutions towards community living – we're trying to unravel the past and we're seeing large institutions gradually disappear, which is a good thing. In the past, it was the common practice for a child with a disability to be put into an institution or "into care", but times have changed. Most children with a disability now live at home. What each family needs is the support and encouragement that should enable them to give their child every opportunity.

'My work involves helping adults with intellectual disabilities to become independent and to lead fuller lives. We also want Ríona to become as independent as possible and we have to be ready for that. She loves to be independent and she is stretching the boundaries for herself all the time. It's difficult to see what her future will be like. If she wasn't deaf, I would see her living independently. I'd hope that would happen, but we don't know really. She might work — perhaps in a restaurant — it depends on whatever her interests might be. We'll have to wait and see. To be honest, work isn't as important as quality of life. Her independence, her quality of life and how she's going to be facilitated in having the choices she'd wish to have are more important than work. I'd hope that she'd be able to live in a house in the community and that she would have the same exposure to everything that anyone else her age would have because whatever fulfils her will be the most important thing. We would prefer not to put the onus on her siblings to look after her; that should not be the case. We would like to ensure that she has some kind of housing in the community. And that is not impossible.'

'That's our project for the next ten years,' says Michael. 'The future is the biggest difficulty that parents have to face and a lot of them ask who's going to look after their child with a disability in ten, fifteen or twenty years time. It's a big worry because it's very difficult to expect the siblings to look after them. I'm sure Ríona's brother and sisters will be very kind to her, but it's too much of a responsibility to expect them to look after her. In bygone days children with a disability were sent to live in institutions — worse still, some were sent to live in psychiatric hospitals — but now the trend is to move people out into the community, which is a good thing. I think the future will be custom-built places of residence provided in every type of community, a bit like sheltered housing for the elderly. You would have a central area where people could get together and you would have day and night staff on duty. I think we have got to see that kind of set-up. I don't see why our child, or anybody else's, should have to leave the place where they've grown up. Parents of children with disabilities must fight to ensure that these kinds of services will be provided in our communities in the future. There's no reason why that can't be done. Why, for example, should Ríona and any other children who have disabilities have to leave Pallasgrean when they reach adulthood?

'The key to the future is people with disabilities living in their community. They have a lot to contribute by their presence: everyone in a community brings their presence and whatever gifts they have. I can see no reason why Ríona shouldn't be a part of everything that's going on in the future in Pallasgrean. She contributes by her presence. Even in church, everybody knows she's there. She troops up to communion and, if people aren't in line, she'll get them into a proper line! They all know she's there and I've never felt that people didn't want her there. They are very accepting.

'We've never found Ríona to be a problem. We have always seen her as a blessing. Of course, if she didn't have a disability, she would be a different person. There's a dynamism in our family and we don't know what it would be like without her — it would be a completely different family. We can't imagine our family without her and we just wouldn't want it to be any different to what it is.'

'What we have I wouldn't change for the world,' agrees Teresa. 'We are very fortunate to have five lovely children — five talented children — each of them very individualistic and with their own special gifts. Having someone in the family with a disability has enriched our lives and has enriched the lives of our other children. I wouldn't have it any other way.'

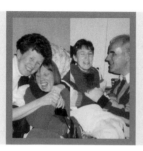

The Hobbs Family

... who refused to despair when Rett's Syndrome turned their lives upside down

'Is it a boy or a girl?' That's probably the first question on the minds of anxious parents following the birth of their baby. Their next concern is to check that their new-born is intact and healthy. Once these facts are established, they can breathe a sigh of relief.

However, some disabilities – even severe ones – are simply not evident at birth. Pat and Anne Hobbs made this unwelcome discovery over thirty years ago. Their first child, Anthony, had entered the world as a perfectly healthy baby and had developed, both physically and mentally, as normal. So, when they were anticipating the birth of their second child three years later they had no reason to expect anything other than another healthy child. Sure enough, when Anne Louise entered the world, on 1 July 1969, she *did* appear perfectly normal. And when she proved difficult to feed and to get to sleep, her parents did not particularly worry. They simply reasoned that babies were different and that they progressed at their own rates.

Their belief was backed up by their GP – even when, at six months, Anne Louise was not sitting up. At her eight-month check-up, when she still had not reached this milestone, they were reassured, once again, that babies differed and that, anyhow, there was not 'a great deal of difference' between the progress of their baby and that of other babies of a similar age.

Anne remembers, 'The doctor popped her on his knee, looked at her and said, "Yes, maybe she is a little bit slow. But if she is a little bit slow, she won't be a complete idiot." I'll always remember those words. He was a good doctor and I suppose he thought he was putting it in a nice way, but it was such a terribly cruel thing to say. I suppose, looking back, we should have known there was something wrong with her, but you go into denial because you don't want to face the reality that there might be anything wrong. And it was devastating to hear that there was.'

They were referred to a paediatrician, who said much the same: 'She's not what she should be for her age.' He saw Anne Louise once every three months, but he never uttered the word that Anne feared to hear. 'He didn't say the word "handicapped"; he just said, "She's not what she should be." He was nice, probably too nice: he never sat me down and said, "Your little girl is handicapped." God love him, I think he couldn't bear to tell me.'

Meanwhile, life in the Hobbs' home in Coventry, England, was exhausting. With Anne Louise apparently unable to do anything other than take short naps, a good night's sleep was impossible to come by. 'It was dreadful because all she would ever do is catnap,' says Anne. 'I don't know how Pat ever managed because the only place she ever found comfortable was on his shoulder. Sometimes he went to work without having had any sleep because he felt guilty if he went to sleep and I was up all night with her.'

Feeding was also an uphill struggle, with Anne Louise finding it difficult to swallow. Mealtimes literally lasted hours on end. 'It was endless because she was taking so little,' says Anne. 'I'd give her a little bit and go off and do something else, then come back and try and give her another little bit. Then I'd have to warm it up and try again. It just went on and on. The reason it was such a struggle was because her throat muscles were affected and she couldn't swallow very well. She couldn't take normal food: everything had to be liquidised and you literally had to try and shovel it in.'

Pat reckons that feeding Anne Louise was one of the most stressful aspects of looking after a child with a severe disability. 'Anne might start trying to give her breakfast at half-seven in the morning,' he says, 'And she'd still be trying to give it to her at ten o'clock. Lunchtime would start soon after that. It just seemed never to end.'

Anne became worn out with the constant feeding and the lack of sleep. 'I felt dreadful,' she says. 'I used to cry for hours — all day and all night — because it was so terrible. I can remember I used to try and pull myself together because of Anthony. He'd be out playing with his friends and he'd come in and look at me and say, "Mummy, don't cry anymore. It will be all right." I'd wipe the tears away, but when he went out I'd look at Anne Louise again and think, "Oh God, no" and I'd start crying again.'

There was no question of Anne returning to her job as a nurse, as she did after Anthony was born. By the time Anne Louise was eighteen months old, she still could not sit up. Neither had she acquired any of the other skills babies are normally expected to have at that age. She did not crawl and, while she did make some noises, she did not babble. Anne and Pat never heard her utter the words, 'Mama' or 'Dada'. Anne says, 'We knew by that stage she was very handicapped, but we kept saying, "We'll be able to do something to help her" and that's why we decided to bring her to London to see a specialist at Great Ormond Street.'

Anne Louise was admitted to hospital for a fortnight, during which time she underwent a series of tests. Pat remembers, 'At the end the consultant sat us down and he really put his cards on the table. He told us that there was a big problem with Anne Louise — that she would never develop very much, if at all, and that she certainly wouldn't develop mentally. That was a shock for us to hear, even though we could see for ourselves that there was something drastically wrong. We had denied it and we had hoped that there might be something we could do.'

Anne continues, 'The specialist told us, "I wouldn't hold out too much hope because I don't think you can expect too much from this little girl." That was dreadful to hear and we left the hospital in a terrible state. On the way home we pulled into a service station and, after we'd had something to eat, I said to Pat, "Right, we're going to accept what's what and you're going to sing again." Pat has a lovely voice and he always used to sing in the house, but I'd noticed he hadn't sung for months. So I said, "You're going to sing again because we're not going to have our house like a mortuary. And we're going to do everything we can for Anne Louise."'

Anne and Pat joined the Association for Brain Damaged Children, which had just been set up in Coventry. 'They were absolutely wonderful,' says Anne. 'We went to their meetings and they gave us great support.'

'They were the first people that ever gave us anything concrete to go on,' adds Pat. 'We knew that Anne Louise needed physiotherapy, but we could only get it on a limited basis. We helped raise funds so that the association could hire a physiotherapist and Anne Louise was one of the first on the list. She certainly benefited from it. The physiotherapist showed us some different exercises we could do with her, which was a big help to us.'

The physiotherapy sessions helped keep Anne Louise's limbs mobile. However, she never gained any skills at all, which was a huge source of disappointment to her parents. With no definite diagnosis, they had nothing to go on. 'It really worried us that, for years, we never had a diagnosis,' says Pat. 'We were always trying to find out, but they would never tell us. You get to a certain level where you accept it, even though you don't know the cause. When you're faced with a handicap, you just have to get on with it — you just do the best you can.'

On entering a third pregnancy, Anne found herself experiencing "dreadful" nightmares. 'I used to dream of two handicapped girls and I said to the doctor, "It won't be another, will it?"'

When Tara arrived on 22 May 1973, she looked perfect – at least, in the eyes of the medical staff. Anne, however, thought differently. 'From the moment she was born I knew she was exactly the same as Anne Louise. I was telling them she was handicapped, but they said, "Look, she's perfect; she's beautiful". Nothing on this earth would convince them that she wasn't all right. But I knew.'

Only when Tara was six months old did a paediatrician agree that, like Anne Louise, she was developmentally delayed. But it was to be another twenty long years before a label was found for the sisters' condition. Rett's Syndrome – first described in 1966 by an Austrian doctor named Andreas Rett – did not become widely known until the 1980s. Caused by a mutation on the MECP2 gene on the X chromosome, those affected appear to develop normally until six to eighteen months at which stage they enter a period of regression, losing any speech and hand skills they may have previously acquired. Most girls (it only affects girls) develop seizures, repetitive hand movements and irregular breathing as well as motor-control problems.

Dr Alison Kerr, who made the diagnosis, reckoned the sisters represented two of the most severe cases she had ever seen. 'I've never seen two as bad as this,' she told Anne and Pat, who have yet to hear of anybody else so severely affected. Whereas most girls have acquired some skills by the time they are affected, their daughters had picked up virtually none. 'We got literature from the Rett's Syndrome Association, which was set up in 1985, and we discovered that a lot of the children could walk and feed themselves before they regressed and lost their skills,' says Anne. 'Our girls are so profoundly affected that they never really had any skills. They never walked, never sat up, never even lifted a toy. It seems our two girls are two of the worst. That's the awful thing about it.'

Although Anne knew straightaway when Tara was born, it didn't make it any easier to come to terms with. In fact, quite the opposite was the case. 'It was dreadful,' she says. 'It was far worse – a complete nightmare – because we were starting the same thing all over again. We knew what was in front of us.'

Anne and Pat quickly realised that they needed to do some serious thinking about their family's future. Looking after one child with a severe intellectual and physical disability was challenging enough, but they knew that to take care of two would be impossible. And there was Anthony to think of, too. They found themselves faced with a momentous decision and it was with great pain and heartache that they began to search for a residential home where Anne Louise could live. They sent away for brochures from homes all over England, Scotland and Ireland. They visited a number of them, including one in Limerick, where Anne is from (they are both Irish – Pat hails originally from Gorey, Co. Wexford). In the end, the best residential centre they found was 150 miles away – near the town of Cromer in Norfolk.

'When we made the decision to send Anne Louise away from home it was the biggest decision we'd ever had to make in our lives,' says Pat. 'One part of us was saying, "We can't handle sending her away". On the other hand, part of us was saying, "Well, she has to go because we have to look after the rest of the family". In the end, we decided that if she had to go we would get the best we could for her. And Meadow Cottage in Norfolk turned out to be the best.'

When Tara was two years old she started attending a nursery for children with special needs, enabling Anne to return to work two nights a week. 'It was very good for me to go back because I was very traumatised,' she says. 'I was devastated after making the terrible decision to send Anne Louise away. Neither Pat nor I got proper counselling – there was no such thing then, really – but my colleagues at work were terribly interested to hear about my daughters and I found, in a way, that talking to them was counselling, for me, because it gave me an opportunity to unload.'

Two years later, Pat and Anne made another momentous decision – this time, to move Tara into Meadow Cottage. 'Anthony was very, very sad when she went away because he was very close to her,' says Anne. 'He used to ask, "Why does she have to go away?" But it was just killing us going up to Norfolk, seeing Anne Louise, and coming back again to the same nightmare we'd already been through.'

It's almost thirty years now since Anne Louise moved into Meadow Cottage. She never did get over her problems with swallowing and, for the past twenty years, she has been fed straight into her stomach through a gastroscopy tube. Tara, on the other hand, has always managed to eat and drink enough to sustain herself. They both receive regular sessions of physiotherapy, hydrotherapy and aromatherapy. Unlike the other residents, however, they receive no speech therapy. There would be no point since they never developed any speech, although they do make some noises and they do manage, to an extent, to communicate with each other.

'In their own way, they certainly chatter between themselves and they answer each other,' says Anne. 'And we know, by their reactions and by the way they turn their heads, that they know us and that they understand every word we say to them. Anne Louise is always smiling and laughing – there's squeals of laughter from her. Whereas Tara is a little lady – she's much quieter and she is very gentle.'

Anne and Pat continue to make regular visits to Norfolk – at least once a month. Anthony does, too. For years Anne feared that he would 'run away' from his sisters, but these fears have turned out to be groundless. 'At the end of the day they are my sisters and, although they weren't at home for many years, there's still a connection because blood's thicker than water,' says Anthony. 'It's obviously a different kind of relationship than my friends have with their brothers or sisters, but I like going to visit them and, after a few weeks, I find I want to see them.'

These days Anthony is joined by his daughters, four-year-old Emily and baby Hannah. 'Emily is fantastic,' he says. 'She just climbs all over Anne Louise and Tara in their wheelchairs and they don't seem to mind at all. It's hard to judge if they're pleased to see us; you wouldn't really know. Sometimes you think you've got a reaction and sometimes you're not quite so sure. I haven't explained anything to Emily, but I'm sure the questions will start in the next couple of years.'

At the births of his daughters, there was a fear lurking in the back of Anthony's mind because he knew Rett's Syndrome had a genetic link.

'Everybody was concerned to see if they were boys or girls, but I just wanted to make sure that they looked around. With my sisters, I don't think their reactions were normal from birth. But, when my daughters were born, I could tell straightaway that they were normal because their head movement was completely different from my sisters'. And that's what I was looking for. Not whether they were boys or girls.'

His parents were tremendously relieved, too. 'For years I was beside myself with worry, not knowing if Anthony was a carrier, worrying that he would pass on the condition to his children,' says Anne. 'That was a terrible time – it was a nightmare – because I carried such guilt, such terrible guilt. We've had so much pain over the years and we were so traumatised and so upset that the girls had to go into residential care because we could no longer cope with them. It was very, very distressful for many years, really, before we could come to terms with it. There's no doubt about it: Rett's Syndrome turned our lives upside down. It took over. Even now, it's still so much a part of our lives.'

With Pat and Anne's families in another country, what has helped them keep going through the difficult times? Firstly, a number of 'wonderful' friends have been supportive and proved invaluable as babysitters. Secondly, a strong marriage has proved an invaluable asset. 'Thank God, it never put a strain on us as a married couple,' says Pat. 'I think sometimes we thought we could talk our problems away. We'd have another mug of tea and another mug of tea and we'd keep talking, which certainly did help.'

Their faith has also helped them keep their heads above water – they are both Roman Catholics. 'I think it was our faith that kept us going,' says Anne. 'I'm just so thankful to God that everything has worked out – that we have been able to see it through together and that He has given us the strength to keep going. We never grew bitter and we just got on with our lives. Even when Tara was born and we were so traumatised, we never got angry with God and we did try to get on with our lives.'

Do Pat and Anne have any advice for other parents of children with intellectual and physical disabilities? 'Join an organisation,' says Pat, without hesitation. 'Because when you join an organisation you get some comfort from the fact that you are not the only ones in that situation. We got so much help from two organisations in Coventry — the Association for Brain Damaged Children and the Catholic Handicapped Fellowship. If you can get up the courage to contact an appropriate association, it will certainly be a help.'

'Get in touch with a group of people with similar problems, so that you can share with each other,' Anne agrees. 'Getting involved in organisations made such a difference to us. People were so supportive and we found that, by getting involved, we didn't feel alone anymore.'

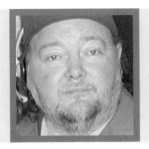

Martin Naughton

... a veteran campaigner who will not rest until people with disabilities enjoy the same opportunities as everyone else

IN MANY RESPECTS, DISABILITY CAMPAIGNER Martin Naughton enjoyed an idyllic childhood in the seaside village of Spiddal, Co. Galway in the late 1950s and early 1960s. He enjoyed exploring his father's thirteen-acre farm and the surrounding area with his brother and six sisters as well as various cousins and neighbours. No one ever let the fact that he had weak leg muscles spoil their fun: whenever necessary, his playmates carried him wherever it was they were going.

'They accepted me the way I was and they didn't seem to mind carrying me about,' recalls Martin. 'It didn't bother them that I rode a tricycle when they were on their bikes and that, past the age of five or six, I had no chance of kicking a football. I managed to walk until I was nine years old, but very poorly: at the age of eight, I probably had the muscles of a two-year-old. Despite that, my memories of life in Spiddal are fabulous because there was plenty to do and lots of places to explore.'

Martin spent two years at the local girls' school, but after that he was expected to move, along with the other boys, to the local establishment for boys. However, this would have been a tougher environment and Martin's parents decided to keep him at home. 'I'd have been happy enough to have gone because, by then, I had already established enough friends who would have protected me,' says Martin, 'But my parents decided it would be too much of a risk because the boys there would have been rougher. I didn't mind at all not going, though, because I had absolutely no interest in schoolwork.'

His parents, however, did mind that he was missing out on an education and, when he turned nine, they decided to send both Martin and his seven-year-old sister Barbara, who also had weak leg muscles, to St Mary's Hospital in Baldoyle, Co. Dublin. He was shocked by the news and the train journey held no excitement for him as he knew it would be a long time before he would make the return trip. 'I didn't want to go,' he remembers. 'Absolutely no way. I really didn't want to go.

'St Mary's was horrible – that's probably the only way I can put it – but there was no support in Spiddal to help my parents cope. We were a big family and my eldest sister, Maureen, who was twenty-five at that time, had the same condition, but it had become very obvious that my rapid progression was much faster than Maureen's had been. She had remained at home, but by that time I was already more disabled than she was. My parents could see it was the same thing, but that I was worse. They were very, very keen on education and they were very, very determined that we would get every opportunity possible and they realised that wasn't going to happen locally. I think it's probably fair to say that the medical profession had a say in the decision, too, because there was a sense that everything possible had been done.'

The fact that Martin only had two years of schooling behind him when he arrived at St Mary's did nothing to help him settle in. And the fact that he had grown up speaking 'as Gaeilge' made it even more difficult for him to fit into an English-speaking environment. 'It was really tough because I had no experience at all of English. The days tended to be very long and kind of sad, especially in the early days, because it was very confusing, not really understanding English. The staff were very nice, but there was huge pressure on them because they were very overworked; it was very institutionalised and extremely crowded. The fact that the staff were nice didn't really compensate for the downsides. I struggled to get a handle on school. I was probably lucky in the sense that I wasn't alone because Barbara was there, too – it was probably harder on her because she was even younger than I was. We were lucky enough in the sense that we got home for a couple of months every summer as well as a lot of Christmases.'

Within a year of moving to Baldoyle, Martin's condition had progressed at such a rate that he could not take more than one or two steps and, following a bout of mumps, he never regained sufficient strength to take even a single step. And so, at the age of ten, he began to use a wheelchair. 'I never had any regrets about not walking again because the struggle of trying to keep going on my feet had been unreal. Therapists usually think it's best to keep trying, but I don't believe that.'

Martin's parents were told he had muscular dystrophy (MD) – a condition characterised by the progressive degeneration and weakening of muscles. 'It was very confusing because the little that was known about MD was that it only manifested itself in boys. They used to say things like, 'Martin definitely has it, but Maureen and Barbara don't because girls can't have it.' It was 1984 before any of us had a definite diagnosis of spinal muscular atrophy, which is part of the same family as MD. They say that it's genetic and that, for it to be inherited, it takes both parents to be carriers. My parents didn't have it, but they must have both been carriers. It affects you from birth, but it really only starts to manifest itself at around three or four years of age.'

Just as Martin was finishing primary school in St Mary's Hospital, a new secondary school opened within yards of the hospital. 'I fitted right in,' he says. 'There was one little technical difficulty, though: it was a school for young ladies! I went there for six years and I enjoyed being the only boy. I loved everything there that had nothing to do with the classroom: being in class was pure hardship and I used to check out of the classroom at every opportunity. I liked the social aspect and I became very involved in netball and athletics. I refereed and gave orders, which came naturally to me!'

During his time at St Mary's, Martin became involved in fundraising for the hospital. 'There was a huge fundraising campaign for years, with people out collecting every weekend. I was knee-high to a grasshopper when I started making lodgements and organising who would collect the following weekend.'

On completing his education in 1972, Martin lived at St Mary's for a further year and managed the newly built swimming pool. 'I had always been more interested in work than I ever was in school: I was interested in anything I could earn a few bob out of. I was particularly interested in recreation work with people with disabilities.'

A year later, he went to live in a newly opened Cheshire Home in Phoenix Park, but continued to work at St Mary's. 'My challenge was to start breaking down the whole routine of the institution. It was a wonderful challenge to get people to feel differently about themselves – to dream a bit and to have a go at whatever they wanted to do. Essentially my role was to focus on recreation – not just on sport, but to introduce other activities, like Scouts and Girl Guides, as well. It was all about opening up the place and bringing in people from the local community. It was integration on our terms and it was hugely exciting.'

By 1981 Martin wanted to move beyond the 'safe' world of St Mary's to find regular employment. 'I started to realise that I needed to see something beyond disability – something that would challenge me – and I needed to take some risks. I saw a house for rent in Baldoyle and I signed an agreement to take it the same day I gave up my job with its pay and pension. Talk about an afternoon of craziness! I decided to get involved in the motor industry – in the area of crash repairs – even though, at the start, I didn't know one end of a screwdriver from the other! It was simply a question of getting stuck in and, within a relatively short period of time, we had a fair market share.'

By 1987 Martin was looking for another change and he spent six months in Boston where he looked after groups of Irish students spending the summer there on JI visas. He met them at airports and arranged accommodation and job interviews for them. For the next few years he spent six months each in Dublin and the US, where he began to feel 'more at home' and where he found people more 'disability friendly'. He was impressed by the Boston Center for Independent Living and, on his return to Dublin, he became 'seriously involved' with the Independent Living Group.

The 'independent living' philosophy is about working for equal rights and opportunities for people with disabilities and is based on the premise that people with disabilities want the same life opportunities and the same choices in everyday life that their able-bodied brothers and sisters, neighbours and friends take for granted. That includes growing up in their own family, going to the neighbourhood school, using the same bus and securing employment that is in line with their education and abilities as well as enjoying equal access to the same services and establishments of social life, culture and leisure.

'The whole goal of "independent living" is to take back control and responsibility for our own lives,' says Martin. 'Where people live is, in some respects, immaterial. The important thing is that they live where they want to live — whether that's in an institution, an igloo or a house doesn't matter. If it's good for them, then it's good. The Dublin group was very energetic and enthusiastic and there were a couple of interesting conferences around that time. People seemed to have the same kind of vision as I had and a group of us went to England and visited Centres for Independent Living in Hampshire, Berkshire and London. By the end of the week we were amazingly enthused and in 1992 we formed the Centre for Independent Living (CIL) in Dublin.

'As a result of the old medical model people with disabilities became very passive and very dependent. It was often a case of "doctor knows best" and the focus was on rehabilitation – putting right what's wrong. That attitude was very undermining because to put right what's wrong means to focus very much on the repair side of things. And the reality of life is that most people can't repair the damages.

'The idea behind "independent living" is to challenge people with disabilities to take responsibility for their own lives. We like to say, 'Nothing about us without us'. Often people with disabilities are not looking for rehabilitation because they don't see anything wrong with themselves; they don't see disability as the nightmare that everybody else seems to see it as. They want to get on with the boring things of life that everyone else is concerned with – work, education, mortgages, transport, social life.

'Sometimes we like to use the term, "Going boldly where everyone else has gone before". We say this to help build up our self-esteem and to encourage a "go-for-it" approach because we are not interested in charity. In fact, we ask people to walk past the can that is being shook in their face as they walk down the street, unless they know exactly where that money is going. We feel that our services should be there as a right – that it should not be a scenario where we are dependent on people's spare change.

'That's all very easy to say, but it seriously challenges people with disabilities to role model that way of living and we need lots of support in order to do that. Although, over the last number of years, we've had a policy of inclusion in this country, it's not enough just to invite people in. People with disabilities have to be supported in order to be able to participate in education, employment and housing. That's one of the big challenges.

'When I operated within the medical model of twenty or thirty years ago, if I didn't succeed, it was my own fault: if I didn't learnt to climb steps or climb aboard a bus – somehow or other, that was my failure. The approach was to rehabilitate; I really was expected to learn to climb steps. The idea was to get people with disabilities to do the things everybody else does and to get them to do them the same way. But today, if I can't climb a bus, society says it's the person who designed it who's got it wrong. That's what inclusion says, whereas integration said, "Stop the bus for him, but if he can't get on it's not your problem". That's the kind of change we've seen in this country.'

Martin cannot find fault with current government policy, but he encounters plenty of problems with its practice. 'You can't fault its policy, really,' he says. 'Through the strategy for equality we set out our goals, but we're now at the stage that it's become cheap talk because there isn't the support for mainstream inclusion. The government has certainly talked the talk, but it's doing absolutely nothing to walk that walk. To me, it seems the government has signed up to something that was only ever going to be possible on a fine weather day, judging by the kind of funding that has been moved into services for people with disabilities. We need some serious front-loading in terms of investment and that really hasn't happened yet.

'When you are a person with a disability you require so many different services – and the more disabled you are, the more services you need. That brings you in contact with a range of service providers – not occasionally, but almost on a daily basis. But if the organisations providing the services start to get nervous about funding, that has a huge effect on the people getting their services. There are a lot of groups that are worried at the moment and I think that's making people with disabilities very nervous and very scared.

'One of the challenges over the last number of years has been to encourage people to have a go, to have a role and to have a life. And the people who did this are now being put off because the confidence isn't there that they will be supported to keep going forward. I think people with disabilities in this country are in a very precarious position at the moment. I'd say they're probably tired now fighting for funding. I think a lot of people feel that, by now, they should just be getting on with their lives. And not still having to fight.'

Since 1997 Martin has been employed by the Disability Federation of Ireland (DFI) – a national umbrella organisation for voluntary non-statutory agencies which provides support services to people with disabilities and disabling conditions. It currently has seventy-five full member organisations as well as having an association with up to two hundred other groups throughout its eight regional networks. Its overall role is to provide a range of supports and services to voluntary organisations that will enable them to deliver the best possible range of services to people with disabilities. Until recently Martin was regional support officer for the entire country, but now there is one support officer for each health board region, Martin taking responsibility for his old stamping ground of north Dublin (he still lives in Baldoyle).

'My role is to bring support to member organisations – to connect with groups at regional local level and to represent them at regional local level. We support them in a whole array of different ways – first of all, by providing them with information on what's happening generally, but also by helping them in terms of representation at all levels – both nationally and at a European level. Basically, my work has involved creating structures at regional and local level where groups can come together and learn about the changes that are going on. I think groups have begun to realise that part of their challenge is to talk to one another, whereas they used to feel they would be stronger if they stayed apart. Now that they are dependent on funding coming from the state, we have to create platforms where they can come together and talk.

'Advocacy and the development of people with disabilities is another big challenge that has almost been ignored. There was a lot of advocacy during the early days of CIL and, when that happened, everything else worked much faster. At the end of the day, we still have a lot happening and, believe it or not, we were a lot poorer ten years ago than we are today.'

Martin believes that the European Year of People with Disabilities is 'a positive thing' and hopes its good effects will reach far beyond the end of 2003. 'I hope it will not be used as a way of taking disability off the agenda,' he says. 'In other words, if people say to us afterwards that the issue has been dealt with, we've had our year, now go away. We have to be careful that the year has some depth to it – that the issues raised can be sustained – because, sometimes, when you really turn the heat up on something people get fed up and end up ignoring the issue.'

Whatever happens, one thing is certain: Martin Naughton will continue to be at the forefront of advocacy and development work. 'Let's not make the mistake that because two or three per cent of people with disabilities live good lives, as I do, that the battle has been won for the remaining ninety-seven per cent. The goal is a simple one: why can't everyone with a disability lead a good life? By that, I mean a life of inclusion and participation – having a home, a job and the same opportunities as everyone else.

'People with disabilities just want to go boldly where everyone else has gone before,' he concludes. 'That's my vision. It's a simple one. And, dead or alive, I'll not rest until that's the case.'

Able Lives CD Track List

1. Scorn Not His Simplicity* –
    written and performed by Phil Coulter
    (Four Seasons Music)

2. Carrickfergus
    – *written and performed by Phil Coulter,
    accompanied by Claire Gallagher* (Four
    Seasons Music)

3. Beethoven's Moonlight Sonata
    – *performed by Claire Gallagher*

4. Aria from Bach's Goldberg
    Variations
    – *performed by Siobhán Keane*

5. A Suite for Siobhán
    – *composed by Philip Martin*
    (copyright Contemporary Music
    Centre, Ireland); *performed by
    Siobhán Keane*

6. Concertino for Piano and
    Orchestra
    – *composed by Daniel McNulty**;
    performed by the RTÉ Symphony
    Orchestra, conducted by Tibor Paul, in
    April 1964*

7. Andante for Strings
    – *composed by Daniel McNulty;
    performed by the Dublin Chamber
    Orchestra, conducted by Herbert Poche, in
    1961*

8. Song for Yona
    – *composed by John Billing; performed by
    the Camphill Community Celtic Lyre
    Orchestra*

9. Spanish Point
    – *composed and performed by Brendan
    Monaghan, accompanied by the Camphill
    Community Celtic Lyre Orchestra*

10. Rose of Allendale
    – *traditional Irish song performed by
    Lughaidh Ó Modhráin*

11. If My Heart Had Wings
    – *composed by Brendan Graham and
    Jimmy Walsh; performed by Lughaidh Ó
    Modhráin*

*   Phil Coulter wrote this song following the birth of his son, who had Down Syndrome

** The late Daniel McNulty (1920-1996) of Rathfarnham, Dublin was a prolific
    composer during the mid-twentieth century. Andante for Strings is an arrangement for
    strings of the second movement of his Divertimento for Orchestra, which won a first
    prize at the Oireachtas in 1957. Blinded in an accident at the age of four, McNulty
    laboriously dictated his compositions note by note to his mother, Josephine, and, after
    his marriage, to his wife, Ann. During an interview on RTÉ Radio in 1958 he
    described his impulse to compose. He said, 'I enjoy walking in the countryside,
    listening to the sounds of nature – singing birds, running streams, whispering trees or
    the peaceful lapping of wavelets by the lake-side. Such pastoral delights create in me
    moods conducive to musical composition. Even though I am blind and cannot see the
    grandeur of scenic beauty or visually appreciate ancient ruins, I can always sense a
    wonderful intangible atmosphere about such places, which I feel I must translate into
    music.'